Oceans of Love

Dear Mum,

I thought this book had an appropriate title, as although I am a long way across the oceans, I am fortunate to always feel loved;

All my love always

xx

25/12/09

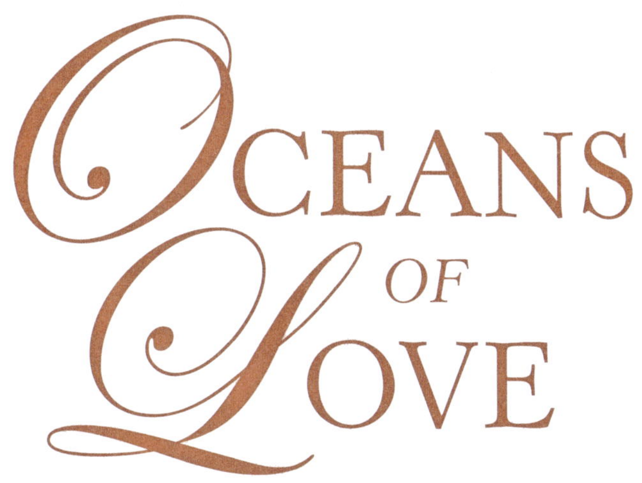

Oceans of Love

Narrelle ~ An Australian Nurse in World War I

Melanie Oppenheimer

For Isabelle,
Lucienne and Camille

Published by ABC Books for the
AUSTRALIAN BROADCASTING CORPORATION
GPO Box 9994 Sydney NSW 2001

First published July 2006

ISBN 10: 0 7333 1710 3
ISBN 13: 978 0 7333 1710 1

Designed by saso content & design
Maps by Ian Faulkner
Cover design by saso content & design
Cover images from the Hobbes Collection
Typeset by 1000 monkeys *in Revival 555 BT 11.5/16pt*
Printed and bound in Australia by Griffin Press, Adelaide

5 4 3 2 1

Contents

List of Abbreviations

AANS	~	Australian Army Nursing Service
AIF	~	Australian Imperial Force
AGH	~	Australian General Hospital
ALH	~	Australian Light Horse
ALP	~	Australian Labor Party
ATNA	~	Australasian Trained Nurses' Association
CWGC	~	Commonwealth War Graves Commission
MO	~	Medical Officer
NAA	~	National Archives of Australia
POW	~	Prisoner of War
QAIMNSR	~	Queen Alexandra's Imperial Military Nursing Service Reserve
RAMC	~	Royal Army Medical Corps
TPI	~	Totally and Permanently Incapacitated
VAD	~	Voluntary Aid Detachment
YMCA	~	Young Men's Christian Association
YWCA	~	Young Women's Christian Association

Acknowledgements

There are many people I wish to thank for assisting me in bringing Narrelle Hobbes' story to life. Rona MacKay, Narrelle's niece, has been very generous over the years in providing many of the essential primary documents, and for sharing her time and memories with me. Victoria Haskins, from another branch of the family, has also been enormously helpful, especially in piecing together Narrelle's family background, and for making available some of the early pre-war photographs. I cannot thank her enough for her friendship, her keen historical mind, and for suggesting the book title. Other family members, such as Tina Withers-Payne and Betty Hall, have both, over time, provided me with additional letters. Betty also gave me the small photograph album from which many of the illustrations have come, and I thank her and her husband Richard for allowing me to reproduce them in the book. I am grateful to Mary Hazelton from 'Narrelle' in Pymble; Barbara and Douglas Webb, the children of Frank Webb; and David and Julia Hardy (Holt Hardy's family) for giving me photographs and information, which helped fill in the gaps. Likewise with Madonna Grehan for her assistance with locating the St Kilda Private Hospital; nursing historians Judith Godden and Kirsty Harris for their interest and knowledge of World War I nurses generally; Peter Stanley from the Australian War Memorial for answering my many brief and not so brief questions; and Anne Marie Condé, also from the AWM, who alerted me to Margaret Hobbes' correspondence with that institution in the 1930s when Narrelle's letters were first donated. Kate Evans and Michelle Rayner from ABC Radio National gave me wonderful support with the radio documentary, which encouraged me to continue with the project in written form. I would also like to thank Lyn Tranter from Australian Literary Management, and Susan Morris-Yates, Commissioning Editor at ABC Books for believing in me and Narrelle's story, and making the book a reality.

Behind every writer stands family and friends. Thanks to my cousins Belinda and George Burnet for their hospitality when I made last minute research dashes to Canberra; to Lindy, Jennifer and Peter Ryan for providing the best writer's retreat at Dungog; to my brother and sister, Martin Oppenheimer and Alex Murray and their families for just being there; and to Bruce Mitchell and Jillian Oppenheimer to whom I am forever indebted. History is part and parcel of our family life and we are all the richer for having such erudite and entertaining parents on tap. My mother is a constant source of inspiration to me, there is simply nothing she would not do for her family, and her spiritual and emotional support is a gift from heaven. No more so than during the long gestation of this book. To Mark, your patience, support and love has sustained and nourished me. I simply couldn't do it without you. And to our daughters, Isabelle and Luci who are becoming talented historians in their own right, thanks for listening and helping me get the life/work balance right; and to Camille, the light of all our lives, who makes us laugh, and will keep us forever young.

Introduction

In the leafy, well-established suburb of Pymble on Sydney's North Shore, just off busy Mona Vale Road, is a quiet suburban street named Narelle Avenue. At the end of that street on the left is a rambling old 1880s weatherboard cottage, one of the original houses in the area. It is set back in a well-loved but slightly out of control and overgrown garden containing a mixture of native shrubs, azaleas and wisteria intersected with stone and pebble pathways. Bordering the garden are oaks, palms and the occasional, absolutely huge, gum tree. The entrance from the street is marked by two gateposts made from blocks of Sydney sandstone, aged by moss and time. Attached to the right-hand side, directly above the mail slot, is an old bronze plaque with the name of the house etched into it in capital letters. The house is called 'Narrelle'. Despite the differences in spelling, both the house and the street were named after Narrelle Hobbes, a sister of one of the original owners. Narrelle, a trained nurse, volunteered for active service during World War I and nursed with the British in Malta, Sicily, Mesopotamia and India.

At the outbreak of war, in August 1914, thousands of Australian men heeded the call to enlist in the Australian forces. Off they went, leaving their homeland for mysterious places such as Gallipoli that most Australians had never heard of before, let alone been able to find on a map. By the end of World War I, in November 1918, over 330,000 men with the Australian Imperial Force (AIF) had fought the enemy on foreign soil. Australian women actively participated as nurses and, while the official figures vary, it is estimated that over 2100 enlisted in the Australian Army Nursing Service (AANS). The motives for these women were similar to those of their male counterparts — they went for the adventure, travel, glory, patriotism and Empire.

For all the women left behind, there was fundraising for the Australian Red Cross and other patriotic funds, knitting and, of course, waiting. Some women wanted more, but their gender stopped them from taking an effective part in the war being fought on the other side of the world. The nature of warfare, the fact that women could not 'bear arms' or be part of a fighting force, and the general position of women in Australian society at the time made it almost impossible for them to do more. Despite these restrictions, many women managed to play a more active role.

Hundreds of intrepid Australian women, including fully trained nursing sisters, took it upon themselves to travel to Europe and enlist. As a result, during the war many did amazing things in obscure and exotic places. This is one of the great ironies of World War I, for, despite all the social and bureaucratic obstacles of the time, Australian women were largely able to go where they wanted. By World War II, restrictions were placed on travel for all non-combatants but this was not the case during the earlier war. Australian women, therefore, worked as nurses, doctors, drivers and canteen workers in Egypt, Palestine, Mesopotamia, England, France, Italy, Burma, India, Vladivostok, Abysinnia, and on transport and hospital ships.

Many, like Narrelle Hobbes, enlisted in the British Queen Alexandra's Imperial Military Nursing Service Reserve (QAIMNSR). Others volunteered their services for the YWCA or the British and French Red Cross as VADs (Voluntary Aids), and worked for little or no pay in the convalescent homes in England, Paris, Rome and Sicily. Some became attached to private and portable hospitals, financed and run by wealthy American and British women, such as Lady Rachel Dudley's Australian Field Hospital in France, or Elsie Inglis' Scottish Women's Hospital in Serbia. The famous Australian author and writer Miles Franklin worked with the American unit of the Scottish Women's

Hospital (under fellow Australian Dr Agnes Bennett) near Salonika for six months in the latter stages of the war. Miles volunteered her labour, so was never paid for her war work — and she caught malaria as a reward. Even the Australian Red Cross sent twenty trained nurses to France in 1916. Called the Bluebirds because of their distinctive uniforms, these 'gifts for France' worked in hospitals and casualty clearing stations attached to the French Red Cross.

In other words, it was an uncontrolled free-for-all. If you had the skills, motivation and nous, you could get to a war zone and contribute your skills and labour in either a paid or unpaid capacity, depending on your circumstances. These Australian women left their country under their own steam and paid their own way, to follow husbands, fiancés, brothers, lovers, cousins and friends to Egypt, and later to London, France or wherever. They undertook active service during the war as nurses, doctors, VADs, fundraisers, canteen operators, and administrators. They have never been properly accounted for or acknowledged, and it is unlikely you will find their names in the hallowed halls of the Australian War Memorial or elsewhere.

NARRELLE HOBBES WAS ONE OF THESE WOMEN. SHE WAS A QUALIFIED nursing sister from rural New South Wales, working as the matron of Brewarrina Hospital when the heir to the Austro–Hungarian empire, Franz Ferdinand, and his wife Sophie were assassinated by Balkan nationalists in Sarajavo in June 1914 — an event which was to plunge much of the world into irretrievable darkness for four years. At the time, Narrelle was about to celebrate her 35th birthday. At above average height, with piercing, twinkling china blue eyes, thick dark hair, and the most beautiful, responsive smile, Narrelle had not married despite having several suitors, and many male friends. She preferred her own financial independence and freedom to the restrictions brought by marriage and children.

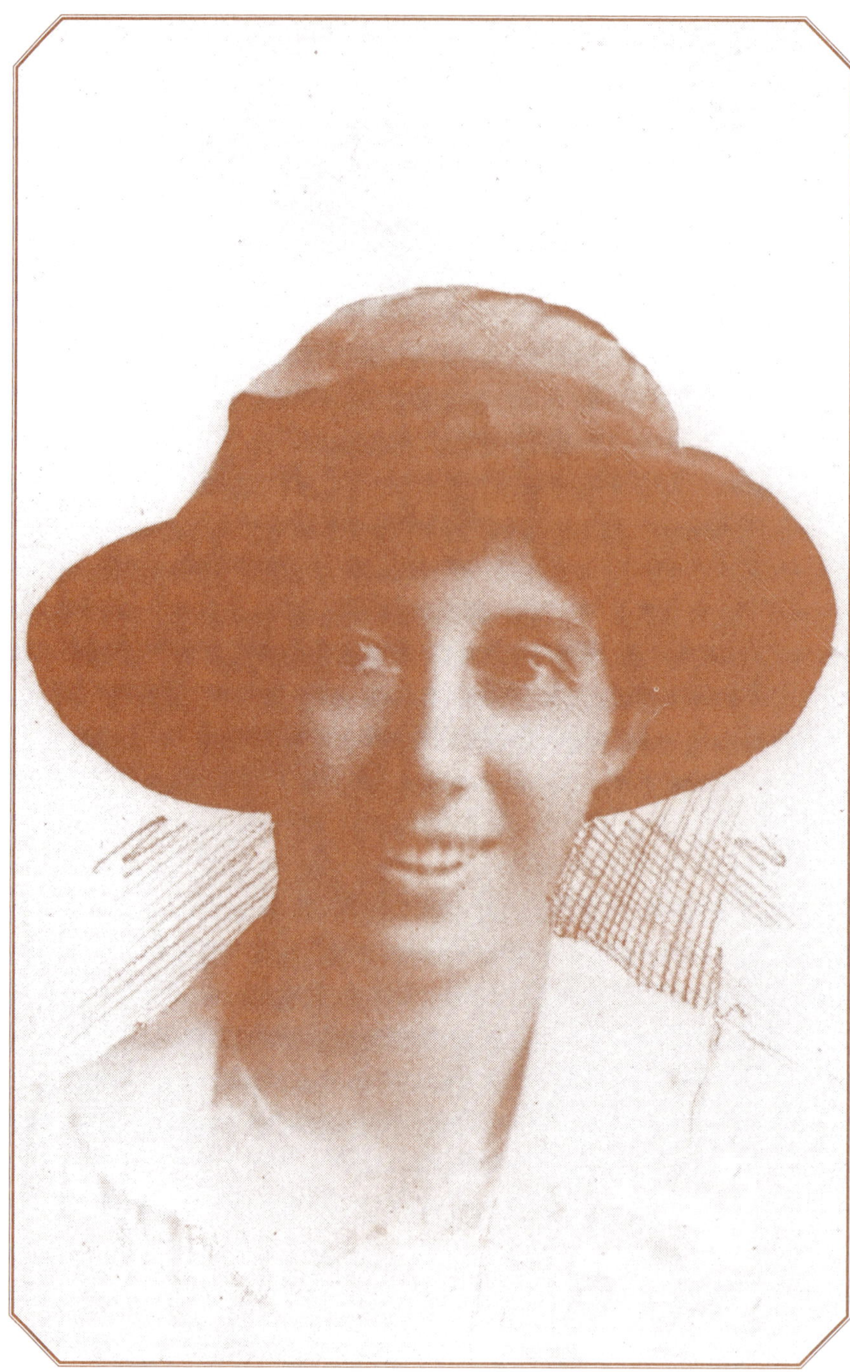

Narrelle Hobbes, circa 1914. (*Hobbes Collection*)

Narrelle was also impatient. Rather than join the AANS, which was not actively recruiting in early 1915, Narrelle headed off, ticket in hand, with a bunch of other girls to nurse for the Empire. She enlisted in London with the British QAIMNSR, and by mid-May 1915 was in Malta up to her elbows in the catastrophe that became known as Gallipoli. Narrelle later nursed wounded and sick British soldiers and officers in Sicily, India and Mesopotamia. By mid-1917, after two years working without respite on active service, Narrelle fell ill and was sent to the Himalayas to recuperate.

FROM THE MOMENT I FIRST HEARD ABOUT NARRELLE'S WAR EXPERIENCES, I was captivated. I cannot remember the exact circumstances, but it was 1991 and I had just given birth to my second daughter and was between jobs when my mother, Jillian Oppenheimer, also a historian, told me Narrelle's story. I immediately wanted to know more, so she introduced me to Rona and Kathleen MacKay, who are nieces of Narrelle's and the only people still alive who actually knew her. Rona, now a sprightly woman in her nineties, encouraged me to write about Narrelle, and directed me to a large collection of Narrelle's correspondence donated to the Australian War Memorial (AWM) in the 1930s by her mother, Margaret Hobbes. These letters cover the early period of Narrelle's war service from London and Malta in 1915–1916, and in Mesopotamia, 1916–1917. Rona then gave me access to a second collection that her mother (Kit MacKay, née Hobbes, one of Narrelle's favourite older sisters) had preserved. These letters covered the period from Sicily and Bombay, 1915–1916, and the Himalayas, 1917–1918. Rona also put me in touch with her cousin, Betty Hall, a great-niece of Narrelle's, and Betty kindly gave me additional letters, a black notebook, and a precious photograph album, the source of many of the illustrations in this book.

I spent months working on the project, transcribing the 70 odd letters onto computer, and trying to pull the material together into a cohesive story. I then received a scholarship to undertake research for a

PhD thesis on civilian volunteers in war at Macquarie University. With great reluctance, I put Narrelle's story aside vowing one day to return. Almost twelve years later, in 2003, with the PhD long completed and another child in tow, I retrieved the precious bundle of files carefully stored away in a filing cabinet.

Once again I was thrilled by Narrelle Hobbes' story, and felt it should be told. My passion was reignited to somehow bring her little-known experiences to the public's attention. A friend, Kate Evans from ABC radio, showed me how I could turn Narrelle's story into a radio documentary proposal, which I took to executive producer Michelle Rayner at the Social History and Features Unit of the ABC, and she commissioned the documentary, 'Narrelle: Nursing for Empire'. I then became researcher, historian and radio producer and spent six months preparing the 52-minute documentary. It included interviews with Rona and principle historian at the AWM Dr Peter Stanley; some dramatisations with my friend, actor Patrick Dickson; and Tracy Mann read from a selection of Narrelle's letters. The program was broadcast in March 2004 on ABC Radio National's program *Hindsight*. It was after this that I discovered another important link for the story. I was contacted by the current owners of the house in Narelle Avenue, Pymble, who had heard the program. All the time I was learning more, and adding to the layers and complexity of Narrelle's story.

Another branch of the family also heard the radio documentary. To my astonishment, a young historian colleague of mine, Dr Vicky Haskins, whom I had met in academic history circles, was related to Narrelle Hobbes. Her great-grandmother, Joan Kingsley-Strack (née Commons) was another niece of Narrelle Hobbes. Joan's mother, Isabel Commons, was Narrelle's eldest sister. It was the Commons who lived in the weatherboard cottage, and named the house 'Narrelle'. Vicky was most helpful and also gave me additional photographs and access to copies of Narrelle's letters held by her family.

Whilst Narrelle did not marry and have children of her own, she had seven siblings and four half siblings so there could be other branches of

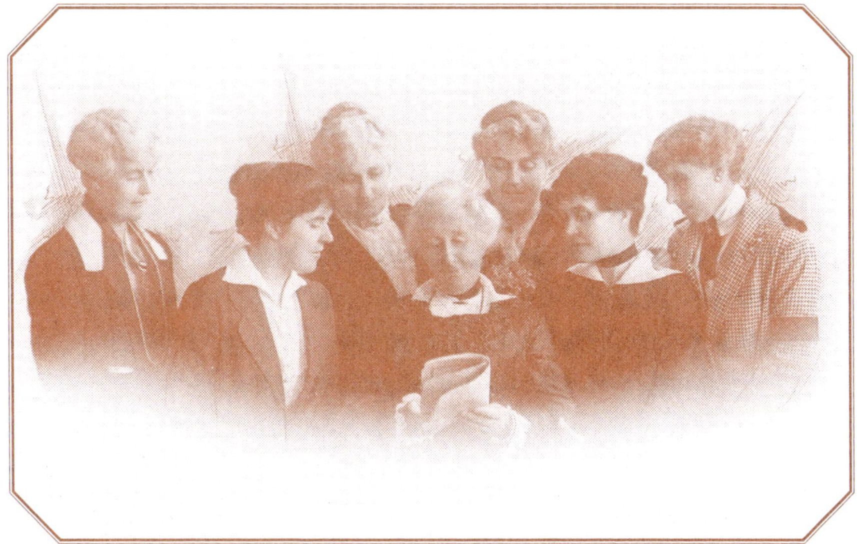

Margaret Hobbes surrounded by her six daughters reading Narrelle's war letters, 1920. From left to right: Kit MacKay, Elsie Hobbes, Isabel Commons, Margaret Hobbes, Jean Magill, Grace Weston and Muriel Weston. (*MacKay Collection*)

the family who may have additional letters, photographs and memorabilia amongst their papers. History is a process of evolution and there are always new ways to tell old stories. So if I have left something out in the following pages, I apologise in advance. Rona MacKay and her niece Tina Withers-Payne from Inverell have continued to produce additional original letters and photographs whilst I completed this project, including the wonderful black and white photograph of Narrelle's mother and her six sisters, taken in 1920.

AS MENTIONED EARLIER NARRELLE HOBBES' WAR STORY IS LARGELY based on a collection of over 90 letters written home to her family in Australia, covering the period March 1915 to April 1918. It is one of the largest and most comprehensive collections of its kind. Many of the letters are originals written in Narrelle's large, open, generous, and accessible handwriting, while others are typed copies. Over the years, other writers such as Katie Holmes, Marianne Baker and Ruth Rae have used extracts of Narrelle's letters from the AWM collection, but they only tell half the story. In *Oceans of Love* the entire collection of Narrelle Hobbes' letters are brought together for the first time. Narrelle also kept a diary but her mother Margaret Hobbes considered it too personal to donate to the AWM. I have been unable to trace it and it may have not survived.

Narrelle did not write her letters for a 'public' audience as such but she wrote them with her large family audience in mind. At the end of one of her letters written in London in early May 1915, she directed her mother to send it on to various family members: *Will you send on to Annie; Annie send on to Charlie; Charlie to Kit; Kit to Nell. I've sent Grace a copy. Nell please return to Mother as she wants to keep them all intact.* After the war multiple copies of her letters were typed and reproduced, presumably so that each family member could have their own set.

To my dismay, when comparing an original handwritten letter with a copy that turned up in another collection, I noticed that there were sometimes subtle changes in the typed version: typographical errors, small sections omitted or changed either inadvertently or deliberately — I am not sure and it does not really matter. I also realised that one of Narrelle's descriptions of the Himalayas from an August 1917 letter, which is very detailed and interesting, was in fact taken word for word from a turn-of-the-century travel book called *Naini Tal Guide of 1906* by Jim Corbett. I was surprised to discover the text on the Internet. There were Narrelle's words — which were really Jim Corbett's words — staring out at me. There is nothing wrong with this in the circumstances. Narrelle regularly bought travel books to inform her about the region she was visiting or working in, and she was not intentionally trying to pass off the descriptions as her own. She was writing privately to her family.

With the above in mind, rather than present a book of edited letters, I decided to create a narrative, weaving the letters into the text alongside my own words. To tell the story of Narrelle's war, her letters are kept separate and distinguished in italics but they are not necessarily distinct letters with a beginning, middle and end. The result is a narrative that flows gently backwards and forwards, almost like a dialogue or conversation between the author and her subject. For this reason, I have also done away with the academic convention of referencing. Narrelle often wrote as she spoke, quickly with few breaks. As a consequence, there are often few full stops, with her letters running on page after page, like a stream of consciousness. I have therefore adjusted some letters for sense and context, adding full stops or breathing spaces where necessary. This was already partially undertaken by family members in the typed letters. At times, too, spelling errors occurred, particularly with place names, and these have also been corrected, for with the typed letters I was unsure whether the errors occurred during the earlier family transcribing or not. All the letters I have used, both originals and typed copies, will be available together as a complete collection in the AWM, Canberra. A full account of the collection is contained at the end of the book in the 'Notes on Sources'.

NARRELLE HOBBES' LETTERS WRITTEN HOME TO HER EXTENDED FAMILY are a witty and evocative reminder of an extraordinary period in Australian history. They explore a range of themes including war, travel, adventuring and Empire from the perspective of an Australian girl from the bush. Narrelle is a real character and this comes through very clearly in her letters home. She is a funny, clever and sometimes formidable woman with a great sense of humour. *Thank God I'm Australian,* she continually wrote as she came up against her British counterparts.

The letters are well written, entertaining, and display a fiery, sometimes intolerant temperament. Like short stories in style and content, they reflect Narrelle's spirited, independent nature and her struggle to come to terms with her geographical and spiritual isolation from Australia and her family — both of which were very important to her. The letters also reveal an impetuous personality who acted on first impressions. Narrelle was judgemental and sometimes highly critical. Sometimes she was racist, reflecting contemporary prejudices and attitudes but she could also change her opinions. Even her dislike and distain of the British — a key theme of her war service in the early years — was later contradicted when she made friends with some of them. Her letters from Malta, Sicily, India, Mesopotamia, and the hill stations of the Himalayas provide the reader with a witty travelogue, with Narrelle, the tourist, in full flight.

Narrelle's letters from Malta show another side of the Gallipoli campaign than the one we have become familiar with in standard histories or documentaries. She nursed the wounded and sick from the peninsula, and through her letters and experiences we learn what happened to soldiers on Gallipoli when they were wounded or evacuated through diseases such as dysentery and enteric fever. The role played by nurses on the hospital ships just off the coast, and at Lemnos, Malta and Egypt is an integral part of the Gallipoli story and Narrelle reminds us that Gallipoli was more than just what happened physically on the peninsula; and that many thousands of soldiers' lives were saved by the medical teams of doctors, orderlies and nurses.

One of Narrelle's motivations for enlisting for active service was to 'help the boys', and the soldiers dominate her correspondence, especially in this early period. Many of her male friends and acquaintances enlisted in the AIF and she met up with some on Malta. Others she regularly corresponded with and often mentioned their exploits or whereabouts in her letters home. A major research task for me was to deduce exactly to whom Narrelle was referring when she talked of Mr Andrews, Frankes, Tonie and Holt, to name a few. I had the painstaking job of searching the army service records — many of which are now, thankfully, digitised on the National Archives of Australia (NAA) website — and the embarkation records from the AWM, for information about Narrelle's friends. For those who died, I also consulted the Commonwealth War Graves Commission (CWGC) website.

Narrelle's war experiences in India and Mesopotamia, too, are especially revealing. The Mesopotamian campaign of 1915 and 1916 between the British and Turkish forces in what is now modern-day Iraq is largely ignored in the war histories, yet the parallels with events today are particularly relevant and of great interest. Narrelle spent nine months on active service working in this sector, one of the most difficult physical environments of the war, with disease and illness rampant.

There has also been little interest in exploring the experiences and stories of nurses in India, an outpost of Empire, during World War I. Yet Narrelle spent seven months tucked away and largely forgotten (by everyone except her family) in the hill stations of India, convalescing from illness. This period resulted in some fascinating letters from her. Narrelle began to reassess her life, and reflect on all that she had witnessed during her active service. She provides us with a unique insight into the mind of a middle-aged Australian women expatriate trapped within the British military system, with little control over her life, but strangely content, surrounded by the physical and spiritual beauty of the Himalayas.

Through the letters of Narrelle Hobbes we can glimpse what it meant to be an Australian woman almost 100 years ago. We can see how women were treated by society, and feel a nurse's frustration at how they were regarded within the military system. We can also understand how Narrelle's war experiences, and her interaction with the British, affected her perception of herself as an Australian. Narrelle became an observer of Empire, a female voice of Australia let loose on the world. She was fiercely patriotic to the British cause but also overtly nationalistic towards Australia. She protected 'her beloved Australian boys' and became obsessed with wanting to nurse them above all others. She travelled to all corners of the British world, from Malta to India — as well as other exotic locations such as Sicily and Mesopotamia — feeling and understanding first hand the exhilaration and tragedy of war. Narrelle Hobbes' story is about one Australian woman's personal journey, and her physical, emotional and spiritual experiences as she found herself propelled across the world during the period of unprecedented destruction that was World War I.

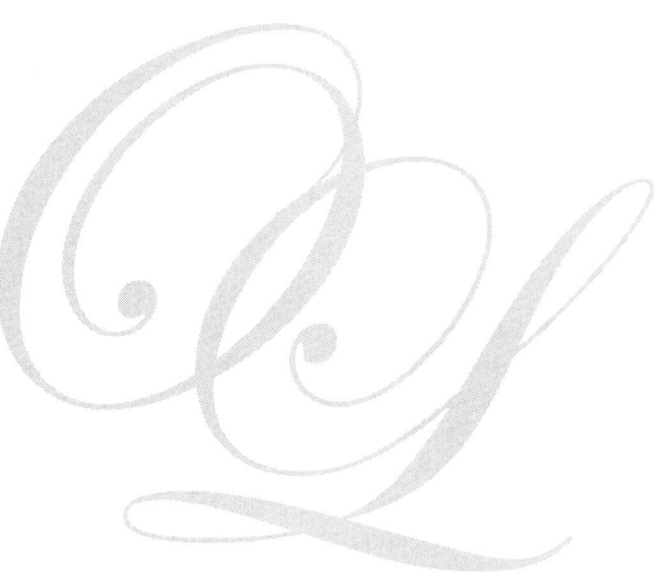

To War

Chapter 1

NARRIE

FLORENCE NARRELLE HOBBES WAS BORN AT 'MERRIWINGA', TILBA TILBA, on the south coast of New South Wales on 21 August 1878. She was never known as Florence, but rather by her second name, Narrelle, an Aboriginal word meaning 'song birds' or, alternatively, 'woman from the sea'. She was named after Queen Narrelle, wife of King Merriman, or Umbarra, an Aboriginal tribal leader who died in 1904. The local Aboriginal people, the Yuin, are the traditional owners of the land around Lake Wallaga, near Tilba Tilba, which became an Aboriginal reserve established by the New South Wales Aboriginal Protection Board in 1891. Narrelle was the second youngest child of her father John T. Hobbes' second marriage. He was 50 years old when she was born.

There are contrasting versions as to her father's origins. In his late twenties, John T. Hobbs (without the 'e') arrived in the colony of New South Wales from London on 28 September 1858. Travelling out on board the *Pam Hush*, as steerage passengers who paid their own fares were John Hobbs and his first wife, Maria Sarah Hobbs née Thomas, the daughter of a wealthy Jewish London jeweller, and their three young children under the age of four. What is not in dispute is that prior to arriving in New South Wales, Hobbs worked for John Ruskin, the famous English writer, author and artist. The question is what he did exactly. Some say Hobbs was Ruskin's secretary and close friend, who travelled extensively throughout Europe accompanying the great man. On meeting the famous English landscape artist J.M.W. Turner in Paris,

Hobbs was given three of his sketches. Hobbs' sister also married George Allen, founder of the publishing house George Allen and Unwin, which published Ruskin's work. This version intimates that the Hobbs' were from the educated, upper middle class. But others argue that Hobbs was a working class Londoner who was Ruskin's valet or personal servant, and whose family worked in domestic service in the Ruskin household. Ruskin was a great believer in working class education and possibly singled out John T. Hobbs as a youngster, took him under his wing, and educated him. This allowed Hobbs the opportunity to travel abroad with Ruskin in a position that today would be called a personal assistant. One of Hobbs' travel diaries written whilst he accompanied Ruskin through France, Switzerland and Italy in the late 1840s is lodged in the Pierpont Morgan Library in New York.

Whatever the reality, and there are probably elements of truth in both stories, as thousands of people had done before him, John Hobbs emigrated to the Australian colonies to find a better life and prospects for himself and his young family, possibly reinventing himself as he journeyed across the world. The family settled in Pitt Street, Sydney, and John Hobbs found a position as the secretary of the Sydney School of Arts. Another child was born and life appeared to be going well for the young immigrants. Sydney was booming. The discovery of gold transformed the colony from merely being a refuge for convicts and their descendants to a thriving and vibrant new society where opportunities for improvement were there for the asking. But tragedy struck on 5 October 1861 when Maria died from complications after delivering their fifth child, Maria Lucy, a month earlier. She left John with five children; John 6, William 4, Annie 3, Alfred 2, and baby Maria Lucy. A month later Hobbs buried his nine-week-old baby daughter alongside his wife in Camperdown cemetery.

Such personal tragedies were, unfortunately, commonplace in nineteenth-century Australia, even though maternal mortality rates were better than in Britain. The death of infants under the age of two was also frequent. Infant mortality was a real and ever present threat. It was not unusual for mothers to lose at least one child under the age of two. Within eighteen months the widower John Hobbs had remarried Margaret Ann Goldie. Margaret (or Maggie as she was known to her family), aged seventeen, arrived in Sydney in 1858 on an assisted passage, with her younger fifteen-year-old sister Euphemia (or Effie) in tow. Their father, Captain Peter Goldie, had worked for the East India Company, and died of cholera just as he was to take up an appointment as a surveyor in Russia at the Imperial Docks. This left his wife, invalided through a childbirth-related injury, at the mercy of her mother and maiden aunts in Dundee, Scotland. Their mother died shortly after their father so the orphans Margaret and Effie were quickly despatched to relatives in Australia. On arrival in Sydney, the two young girls were met by their uncle Captain Robert Stobo and his sister, Mary Waugh, with whom they went to live. Captain Stobo lived near the water at the grand Darley House in Millers Point, and Aunt Mary had a large home in Macquarie Street near the corner of Bridge Street, Sydney.

The opportunities for unmarried middle-class girls of limited financial means and with few prospects were much greater in the colonies than in Britain. With the gender balance clearly in a woman's favour in the Australian colonies, it did not take long for Margaret to make her match. While working as a governess at Woollahra, Margaret met John Hobbs at the Congregational Church where she was the Sunday School teacher. Margaret Goldie and John Hobbs were married on 11 March 1863 at the Kiama Presbyterian Church with Effie and uncle Robert Stobo as witnesses. She was 21 years of age, and John, 35. The newly wed couple, with the four children, moved to Tilba Tilba where Hobbs had selected land under the Robertson Land Act (or Crown Lands Alienation Act) of 1861. Due to the rugged terrain, the main form of transport to and from the south coast was by boat. Hobbs hired a small boat packed to the rafters with all the necessary goods and supplies required by new settlers and sailed down the coast to establish their new home.

Within twelve months, Margaret gave birth to her first son, and John's sixth child. In an extract from her diary (of which only remnants survive) on 1 April 1864, Margaret described her joy at Robert P. Goldie's arrival.

> *What a harvest of mercies I have reaped since I last wrote in my journal. I am now a* real Mother. *Yes our dear boy came to us on the 23 March. How my heart thrilled when I heard his cry. All the pain felt was gone, to be remembered no more … I hope I shall not tire him talking about my boy. I sometimes forget that it is not his first, but he loves me so very very much.*

Tragically, Robert was to die two weeks before his second birthday. He was buried in the Presbyterian section of the Moruya cemetery. Margaret and John went on to have a further eight children, all of whom survived well into adulthood. Not unusually for women of the nineteenth century, Margaret spent much of her twenties and thirties either pregnant, lactating, nursing or weaning infants. Charles Goldie Spence arrived on a cold winter's day, 4 August 1865, and then the Hobbes (at some point an 'e' was added) were blessed with seven girls in rapid succession, nearly all of whom, like Narrelle, were not known by their first names. First there was Isabel Helena Dymock on 20 October 1867; then Mabel Janet Nott (Jean) on 25 June 1869; Margaret Ethel Kate (Kit) on 1 March 1872; Effie Constance Muriel (Muriel) on 24 January 1874; Roberta Grace Dymock (Grace) on 29 September 1876; Narrelle; and last of all Caroline Elsie May (Els) on 4 March 1882.

NARRELLE GREW UP WITHIN THIS LARGE, BUSY, NOISY, CLOSE-KNIT, female-dominated household at 'Merriwinga', the timber house built by her parents near the foot of Gulaga, or Mount Dromedary, charted and named by Captain Cook in 1770. From the house, set high on a hill above Lake Wallaga, one could see the Pacific Ocean to the east and Gulaga towards the west. Trips to Narooma, the seaside fishing village not far away, were sometimes undertaken by the Hobbes family, as it was from there that locals took the boat to Sydney. There is a story about Narrelle who, as a small baby, was taken to Sydney with her parents on the local coastal steamer when it ran into a fierce storm. Pushed by an offshore wind, the boat almost ended up in New Zealand. After days of rough weather, all the crockery, including Narrelle's glass nursing bottles, had been smashed. A quick-thinking crewmember, trying to pacify the screaming infant, ingeniously created a feeding bottle by using a gunpowder flask topped with a finger of a glove. Thus Narrelle, at a very early age, became acquainted with two features that were to play a key role in her destiny — the military and the sea.

Life for the Hobbes' children was free and uncomplicated. They played with the local Aboriginal children from Lake Wallaga, listening to the stories about how the lake was created and other legends. They learnt about fixing cuts and bruises with spider-web threads or the liquid from fern fronds. Perhaps this was where Narrelle first developed her interest in nursing. Fish were caught in the lake and sometimes, if the tide was out, they collected oysters as a special treat. All the children learnt to ride horses at an early age. They were schooled at a little local bush school that was reached by sailing across the lake in a small skiff. Later, the younger children were taught by a governess. And each Sunday the entire Hobbes family — mother, father and the twelve children — would trudge over the lush green hills to the neighbour's farm for a church service. Resplendent in their Sunday best, the older boys carried a small harmonium slung between two poles on their shoulders, so that their beautiful, charming and musically talented stepmother, Margaret, could play the rousing hymn music while the rest of the makeshift family congregation sang.

This idyllic rural childhood came to an abrupt end when Narrelle's father suddenly died, aged 63. In order to secure additional income other than that from the farm and to support his large family, John Hobbes had secured a position as police magistrate at Port Macquarie. He died there, of stomach cancer, on 25 May 1892 after an illness of three weeks, and was buried in the Church of England cemetery.

Narrelle was thirteen years old when her father died. Although Margaret Hobbes went on to buy more land around 'Merriwinga' and became quite the landed matriarch, money was always tight. While her stepchildren were well into their thirties, Margaret still had six unmarried daughters on her hands, ranging from 23 to eleven, with only her eldest, Isabel, having married the civil engineer and artist Donald Commons. The prospects for young middle-class women at the turn of the century largely revolved around marriage and children. The professions were limited to teaching and nursing. The University of Sydney accepted women students but only the bravest and more forceful women could challenge society's conservative conventions. There was also the custom of at least one daughter staying on at home to be their mother's companion, a role that Elsie would play for a time.

Narrelle often stayed with her eldest sister, Isabel, in Sydney, where she was sent to school. By that stage, Isabel had two young daughters, Joan and Helen. Joan Commons (known as Ming) later became a well-known activist against the removal of Aboriginal children from their parents in the 1930s, and an advocate for Aboriginal citizenship. During the 1880s, Isabel's husband, Donald Commons, was employed on the construction of the North Shore railway line, and had bought a 5-acre property near Stoney Creek Road (now Mona Vale Road) in Pymble. The area was covered in thick bushland with mahogany, jarrah, turpentines, and other types of gum trees in abundance. Even today, one can imagine the seclusion and beauty of the place that has retained its fair share of precious bushland. The house was a modest timber cottage with a galvanised iron roof, cedar doors and verandahs, and beautiful wisterias and white banksia roses adorning the garden.

One by one Narrelle's older sisters married and left home. She was particularly close to her second-eldest sister, Jean, a quiet, kind and gentle soul whom everyone liked. Her family nickname was 'the little Missus' due to her resigned domesticity and ethereal disposition. She married a blustery, larger than life Irishman, George Magill, who was the total opposite to his wife in every way. People found him humourless and dictatorial. In 1910, Magill, in partnership with his brother and two brothers from a local family called MacKay, bought 'Weilmoringle', a huge property in north-western New South Wales near the Queensland border, north of Brewarrina. Narrelle would spend much time there before the outbreak of war, just as she would at 'Gunyerwarildi', the Warialda property of Donald MacKay, one of Magill's partners, who married Kit Hobbes. The next two sisters, Muriel and Grace, married the Weston brothers, Charles and Jack respectively, and Grace moved to Tombellup in Western Australia.

The Hobbes sisters appeared to get on with each other reasonably well, which is somewhat surprising given the size and complexity of the family. Their relationships revolved around their strong matriarchal mother who was both the magnet and conduit for the siblings' relationships. While their brother Charlie had the best of both worlds, being the eldest (of their family at any rate) and a boy, Isabel was the eldest girl so that gave her a natural seniority. Everyone loved Jean and it was to her they turned for comfort and reassurance. Kit and Muriel, right in the middle of the pack, were realists and generally just got on with

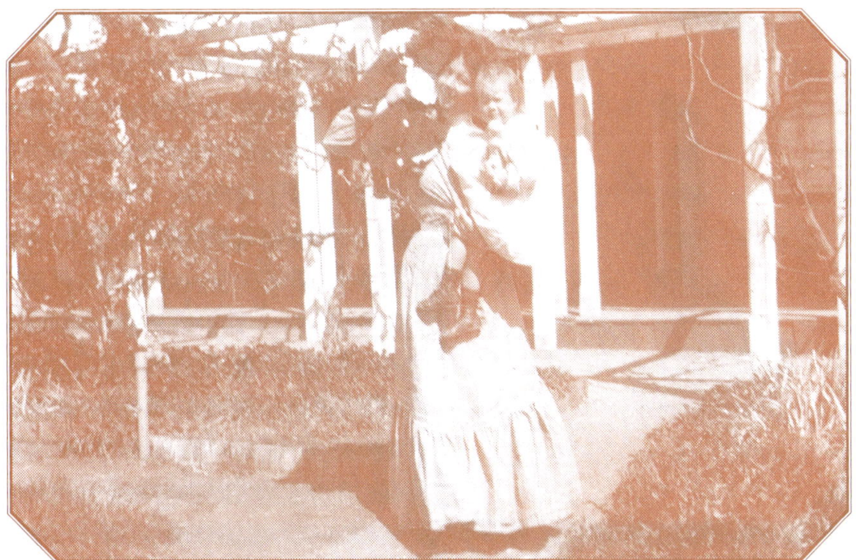

Narrelle and two of her nieces before World War I. (*Haskins Collection*)

things. Grace had the looks; she was stunningly beautiful. Elsie was the baby whom everyone adored. Narrelle was the tomboy, the carefree, wild one, who displayed an innate spirit and *joie de vivre*. As the second youngest, she was virtually brought up by her older sisters, which had its advantages as her parents were too exhausted and preoccupied to try to control her. Narrelle was certainly not willing to conform like her sisters by marrying as expected. She did not discount the eventuality of marriage and children, but she wanted more out of life beforehand. Narrelle decided to take up nursing as a career.

NURSING AT THE TURN OF THE CENTURY IN AUSTRALIA WAS A PROFESSION still in its infancy. The creation of the Australasian Trained Nurses' Association (ATNA) in 1899 was part of the process of professionalisation. Women from the middle and lower middle classes were encouraged to take up nursing in an attempt to shake off the 'Sarah Gamp' image of nurses as the gin soaked Dickensian character with suspicious morals from the novel *Martin Chuzzlewit*. Almost all of the Australian nurses who went to the Boer War, fought from 1899–1902, were considered 'ladies', coming from backgrounds not dissimilar to Narrelle's. Nursing was an appropriate profession for educated, genteel, refined women. However, it was always very badly paid and working conditions were tough. Nursing was a physically demanding job involving long hours carried

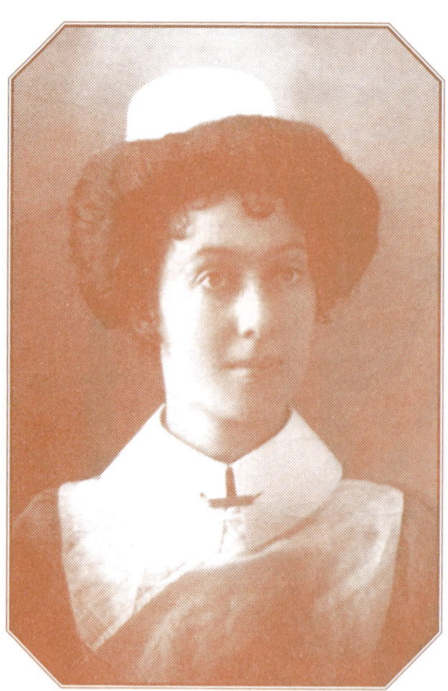

Narrelle Hobbes as a young nurse in her early twenties. (*Hobbes Collection*)

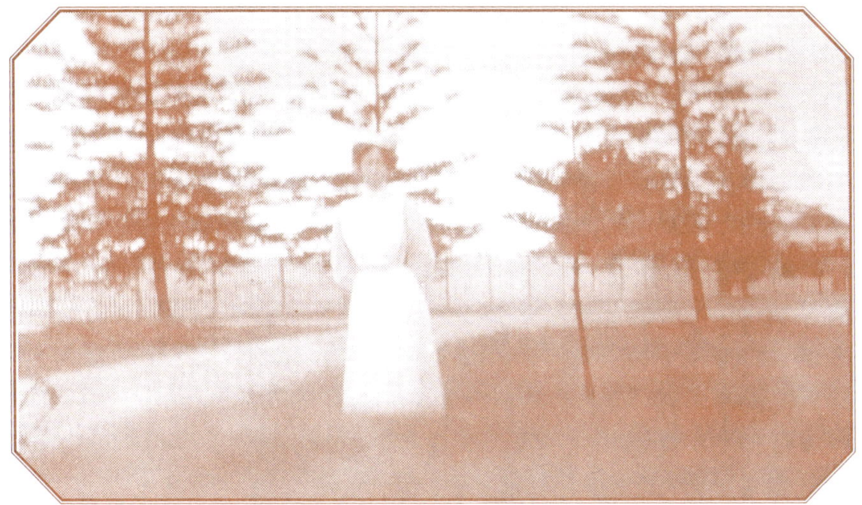

Narrelle Hobbes, Matron of Brewarrina Hospital, 1914. (*Haskins Collection*)

out within a rigorous, rigid and hierarchical environment. But it could also be very rewarding. Through training as a nurse, Narrelle could be financially independent and not have to rely on marriage for security. It also provided an excuse to leave her mother's side.

In April 1903, at 24 years of age, Narrelle began her five-year training course at the St Kilda Private Hospital in Wooloomooloo, Sydney. In New South Wales, private hospitals with a daily average of ten to twenty occupied beds were entitled to provide nursing training. Narrelle trained at the St Kilda for two years until February 1905. For unknown reasons, she then took leave from the St Kilda, returning in March 1907 to continue her training at the Cobar District Hospital in western New South Wales. Narrelle passed her ATNA exams in June 1910, became a member of the ATNA, and was promptly promoted to head nurse at Cobar from July the same year. She held this position until April 1911 when she was offered the matron's position at the equally small and remote Brewarrina District Hospital to the north, which was close to 'Weilmoringle' where her sister Jean lived.

In 1913, Narrelle took leave from Brewarrina Hospital and rushed to Kit's side where there was a medical emergency at 'Gunyerwarildi'.

Her small daughter Rona, only two years old, had contracted diptheria, a highly infectious and potentially deadly disease for children, and was gravely ill. Rona who is a very healthy, active 90-something today, clearly remembers her Aunt Narrie, as she was known to her nieces, as a 'calm, kind, confident presence', a person who gently nursed her back to health. Before returning to Brewarrina, Narrelle assisted her mother and Elsie to move from 'Merriwinga' to Sydney. With most of her children married and living far away from Tilba Tilba, the octogenarian and grandmother Margaret Hobbes decided it was time to pack up and relocate to 'Balblair', a large house in Milson Road, Cremorne, where she would live until her death in 1934.

With her mother settled, Narrelle returned to Brewarrina in March 1914. She always preferred the bush and its people to the city, and she came to love the western plains. Her circle of friends included the Anglican Brewarrina Bush Brothers, Leo Andrews and Wilfred Hartridge, both Londoners. The Bush Brothers, established by the Anglican Church in the first decade of the twentiety century, sent young priests to remote rural areas. Narelle particularly liked visiting 'Weilmoringle', where the social life was legendary. George Magill liked to have young women visiting the property to socialise and play tennis with the jackaroos. As his wife had many sisters, young nieces and their friends, this was never a problem. Narrelle often spent her days off at 'Weilmoringle', riding, picnicking and playing tennis. One such tennis party, in the autumn of 1914, not long after Narrelle had returned to Brewarrina, was captured on camera.

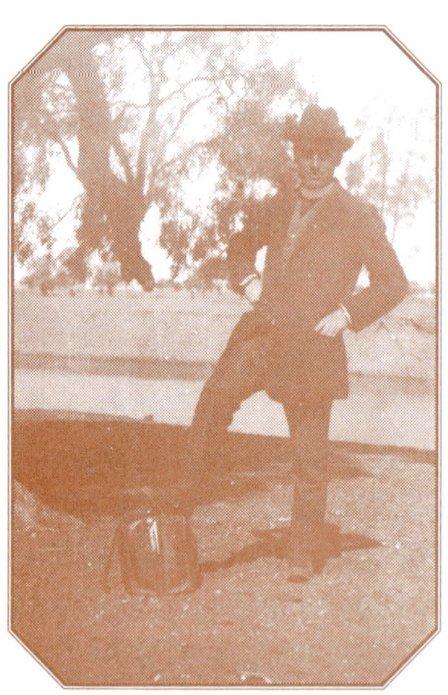

Leo Andrews, a Bush Brother from Brewarrina, 1914. (*Haskins Collection*)

A grainy black and white photograph reveals a group of young men and a woman relaxing after playing a game of tennis. Narrelle, a keen photographer, is possibly behind the lens. The group is sitting just inside the tennis court behind the umpire's chair. A disused water wagon is directly behind the high fence, which is made of chicken wire and thin wooden posts. Tennis racquets are propped up casually against the wire or thrown down onto the dusty ground. The group is sitting on wicker chairs and one is on a wooden fruit box. One boy, in white shirt and bow tie, is skylarking with the woman (Narrelle's niece Joan Commons), standing behind her, perhaps holding the chair for her to sit down. She clutches her cream hat protectively over her head, largely obscuring her face from the camera. The man to their left looks on at the pair, left ankle resting casually over his right knee. A third leans back laconically in the chair, his hat pushed back off his head, with a broad, friendly smile, looking directly at the photographer. He is not dressed for tennis, wearing elastic-sided boots and dark suit and tie. To his left, sits another, shirt sleeves rolled up, hat pushed forward, leaning towards the camera, hands resting between his legs, brown forearms on his thighs.

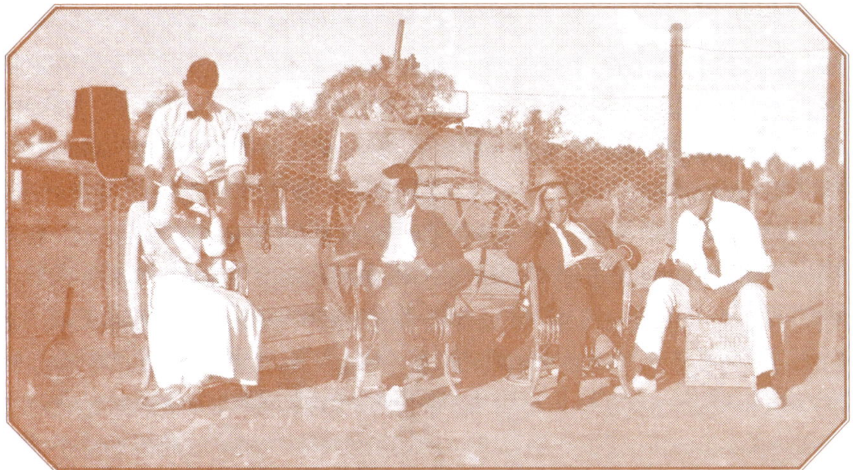

A tennis afternoon at 'Weilmoringle', 1914. From left to right: Joan Commons (Narrelle's niece), Bret Allport, Holt Hardy, Frank Webb and James Langwell. (*Haskins Collection*)

The mood is relaxed and informal. Everyone appears to be enjoying themselves. They are young, happy, vital, their futures yet to be determined. The men were all jackaroos on the property, mostly from the city. From left to right are Roland Bret Allport (always known as Bret), aged 21 from Sydney; Holt Hardy, also 21, born at Homebush in Sydney; Frank Webb, 24, born in Wellington (his father was Inspector of Railways); and James Langwell, the youngest at twenty, also from Sydney, born at Marrickville. In just a few short months, their lives would change dramatically. Their carefree smiles would be lost to the horror of war.

THE ANNOUNCEMENT OF WAR ON 4 AUGUST 1914 CHANGED AUSTRALIA forever. The reaction of the Australian people to the declaration of war was phenomenal. Thousands of men, the cream of Australia's youth, rushed to enlist in the first few weeks of August. Wilfred Hartridge, who according to Narrelle *was such a dear soul, & only a boy, most awfully shy till he got to know you, and then he was awfully amusing* immediately left Brewarrina to enlist. The Bush Brothers wanted him to enlist in the medical services but that did not appeal to him. Hartridge preferred the infantry and enlisted in the 3rd Battalion of the AIF. Jackaroos from 'Weilmoringle' also decided to enlist straight away, and others would follow later. Some, like Cecil Anthony Hordern, always known as Tonie and one of Narrelle's friends, received a telegram from his father Cecil Hordern, a descendant of the famous Sydney retailers, Hordern and Co, declaring that the war was on and asking whether his son wanted to enlist. Tonie answered his father's call, put in his resignation, and headed straight for Sydney, taking a 'Weilmoringle' horse with him to enlist in the 1st Australian Light Horse (ALH). Holt Hardy was also given a station horse when he enlisted in the 6th ALH in September. Another, Ted Nott, rather than join the AIF, headed straight to England to enlist in the King's Own Yorkshire Light Infantry, an alternative route to war. In all, fourteen jackaroos and station workers from 'Weilmoringle' alone enlisted in World War I, including all four men in the tennis party photograph.

From her small hospital in western New South Wales, Narrelle watched all this activity with envy. She was very keen to do something tangible, to make a difference, to join the boys in this great adventure unfolding before her eyes. She did not particularly want to join the home front war effort of 'Red Crossing' and knitting socks, the main options open to women. She knew the value and worth of voluntary work as her mother and sisters were already involved in the Australian Red Cross Society, the fledgling philanthropic organisation formed in Sydney and other states in August 1914 by the wife of the governor general, Lady Helen Munro Ferguson. A close family friend, Mrs Eleanor MacKinnon, was to become a prominent figure in Red Cross circles, founding the Junior Red Cross and editing the *Red Cross Record*.

As an experienced and qualified nurse, Narrelle had the key practical skills required. Military nursing was something that she could do, and there would be a demand in Britain for nurses. Narrelle did not seriously consider enlisting in the AANS nor was she on the nursing reserve list. The AANS was slow to react to the outbreak of hostilities, and there was a perception early on in the war that it was not well organised or managed. While the first two contingents of Australian nurses with the AANS left Sydney in November and December 1914, there were hundreds of nurses waiting for vacancies to occur. As early as September 1914, *The Australasian Nurses Journal* was suggesting to its members that another way to enlist for active service was to travel directly to London with the hope that, as they were on the spot, they would have a better chance of securing work with the British military nursing services.

Then Narrelle's sister Grace Weston, in Western Australia, had a bright idea. She wrote to her friend, nursing sister Miss Birt, who happened to be working in England at the outbreak of war and was now in charge of the huge 2000-bed Red Cross Hospital at Huntingdon, north of London near Cambridge. Grace inquired of her friend about possible options for

Narrelle. Miss Birt responded positively, writing that there were many opportunities for energetic, trained nurses in England. She then wrote a letter directly to Narrelle around Christmas explaining the situation if she wanted to travel overseas and try her luck in London. She also offered Narrelle a job at Huntingdon if other opportunities fell through. It all sounded wonderful. The only thing putting Narrelle off was money, or lack of it. She could not afford a passage to England.

Over Christmas, Narrelle's future was decided. With financial assistance from the family, Narrelle would travel to England and, if nothing else eventuated, take up Miss Birt's offer of work. It was simply too good an opportunity to miss. The war had created a demand for nurses with her skills and experience, even if the sceptics said that she, and others like her, were just chasing rainbows. What would happen if she travelled all the way to London and then could not get work, the doubters asked. What if Miss Birt's offer fell through? Wouldn't being a colonial disadvantage her? What if Australian training was not up to scratch? Was there really a need for so many nurses? Why would they choose her? Should she travel unaccompanied? All these questions, all these doubts were put to one side. If Narrelle was going to make a difference, she had to take the risk. And she had Miss Birt's offer to fall back on.

In January 1915, it was difficult to join the AANS, as others had found. Rose Kirkaldie, for example, who sailed with Narrelle to England and later wrote about her war experiences in the book *In Grey and Scarlet,* was one of the first Australian nurses sent on 'active service'. At the outbreak of war, she was part of a small contingent of seven nurses who volunteered to serve on the *Grantala,* Australia's first hospital ship. Sent immediately to assist with the fighting in German New Guinea, they returned to Sydney in December 1914, and the nurses were discharged. Largely due to disorganisation amongst the medical authorities in this early part of the war, it was thought that no more AANS nurses were required. So there were no more opportunities for Rose Kirkaldie. Her service on the *Grantala* was also not recognised by the military authorities, and she had to re-apply for the AANS. To add insult to injury, Rose found out that she had missed the first contingent of AANS nurses who had sailed with the AIF in November; and the larger group of 161 nurses who had steamed out of Sydney Heads on the *Kyarra* on 5 December to form the 1st and 2nd Australian General Hospitals (AGH). This contingent was made up of nurses on the reserve list and many others hurriedly recruited while Rose was in New Guinea, and Narrelle, Brewarrina.

Like Narrelle, Rose was impatient. She simply could not wait for the Australian medical authorities to recruit more nurses. At this point, there seemed little difference in whether one joined the Australian or British nursing service. The one objective was to volunteer, to serve, to be part of the great adventure, to get to the other side of the world where all the action was, to become active participants like the men. So Rose persuaded her best friend and nursing companion, Elsie Welman, to join her in travelling to London to enlist there. And Narrelle resigned from Brewarrina Hospital, packed her bags and, like many of the young men around her, headed off to Sydney.

Once decisions were made, the next step was to secure a passage on a ship to England. This was easier said than done. From the beginning of the war, shipping had been disrupted and many ships were requisitioned by the Australian and British governments as troop carriers, hospital ships and as part of the general war effort. There were also hundreds of people, including families and reservists, who wanted to return to Britain. The result was long waiting lists and a shortage of berths. Narrelle had to cool her heels in Sydney, and stay with her mother and Elsie in Cremorne, waiting until a suitable and not too expensive berth came up.

The SS *Ballarat* answered her call. The *Ballarat* was part of the P & O shipping line which plied the relatively lucrative England–Australia route, as did other shipping lines such as the White Star, Aberdeen and Blue Funnel Line. Built in 1911, the *Ballarat* offered a one class (or third class) passage for 490 passengers that provided a passable level of comfort. The *Ballarat* was later requisitioned by the British government and sank in the English Channel after being torpedoed on 25 April 1917 carrying Australian troops to France. No lives were lost.

It was very expensive to travel to England. Fares ranged between £16 and £20 one way on a third class ship, to £45 and up on a Blue Funnel Line in first class. Narrelle's sister, Grace, who felt responsible for initiating the idea, paid Narrelle's fare. Even a third class berth on the *Ballarat* would have been almost a quarter of her yearly nursing salary. Narrelle also had to take sufficient money with her to live on if work was not readily available when she reached London. So all the family pitched in where they could and provided either financial assistance or helped with their sister's nursing kit. With brother Charlie, born in 1865, too old, and a family of seven girls, Narrelle was to be the Hobbes' contribution to the war.

ON THE MORNING OF SATURDAY 20 FEBRUARY 1915, WITH STREAMERS fluttering in the breeze, Narrelle made her final farewells to her family at the Central Wharf, Millers Point. It was a typical Sydney February day — hot and sultry with the chance of afternoon thunderstorms. On that day, out on Narrelle's beloved western plains, temperatures of well over 100 degrees Fahrenheit (38 degrees Celsius) were recorded at Narrandera, Balranald and Hay. It was hot, dry, windy, thunderous late summer weather. The newspapers reported that the ship was full to capacity and included volunteers for the King Edward's Horse regiment and nurses for active service. The *Ballarat* was also carrying a significant cargo worth upwards of 1 million.

As the ship quietly slipped its moorings and allowed the tugs to push it away from the wharf, the level of excitement, mixed with trepidation, rose. This was Narrelle's first trip overseas, and she was doing it on her own, all alone, unchaperoned. In fact she had never before been out of

New South Wales. She stood on the deck waving as the ship slowly moved up the harbour, past where the Harbour Bridge and Opera House now stand. Past Cremorne Point on the left-hand side where her mother and sister lived; past Taronga Zoo, swinging left around Bradley's Head. Then the *Ballarat* left the ferry route to Manly, and with a right turn cruised through the Heads and away. The ship slowly turned right and sailed down the coast past the Sydney beaches of Bondi, Tamarama, Bronte, and Maroubra. Narrelle stayed on deck watching the distant coastline until darkness forced her inside.

She soon befriended Rose and Elsie, as well as Sylvia Bell and Kathleen Fitzpatrick, all nurses bound for London. Even today it is unclear how many Australian women served abroad on active service during the war. The official historian of the Australian Medical Services, A.G. Butler, put the number of AANS embarking from Australia at 2139 with an additional 129 officially seconded to the British in 1915 (these nurses were largely sent to India). But there were over 500 more Australian women who have never been accounted for, who served independently of the Australian government in various theatres of war. The Australian government was aware of the trend. In early 1915, the director general of the Medical Services of the Commonwealth, Colonel Featherstone, warned the peak nursing body in New South Wales, the ATNA that many Australian nurses were 'turning up' in England hoping to secure military appointments with little success. Nurses had to have at least three years training in a large public hospital, and were required to be aged between 25 and 40. They also had to have sufficient documentation, such as a sealed reference from their matron verifying full general training.

But these sorts of official warnings had little effect and did not deter adventurous and independent Australian women like Narrelle, Rose, Elsie, Sylvia and Kathleen. They had made up their own minds and were on their way to active service.

Chapter 2

'My dearest people'

On leaving Sydney, the weather deteriorated rapidly, and the run down to Melbourne was rough. 'Dull, windy and wet weather' characterised Narrelle's Melbourne stay with unseasonally chilly temperatures of 65 degrees Fahrenheit (18 degrees Celsius). But the damp and grey skies did not put her off; Narrelle loved Melbourne. She was indulged by cousins who showered her with kindness, and showed her the sights including St Kilda and a trip on Melbourne's famous trams.

The first letter from Narrelle's collection is written from Adelaide on the 1 March. She was still acclimatising to ship life and finding her sea legs. She was also getting used to the crowded nature of sea travel in third class accommodation. There were over 450 people on board, including many children who continually disturbed her. One of her special pleasures was to sit in her deck chair, supplied courtesy of the Australian Red Cross Society, in the fresh air, as it helped keep seasickness at bay. In what would become her signature style, Narrelle began her first letter to 'My dearest people', and signed off with 'Oceans of love, Narrie'. Narrelle described, in effusive detail, the wonderful city of Melbourne in 1915.

> *... I think I've pretty well seen Melbourne from one end to the other thoroughly, and am quite in love with it, the streets, most of them are beautiful and trees growing along each side, plane trees growing to an immense size, forming perfect avenues in places. The footpaths are very*

wide and mostly have no covering like we have in Sydney, and instead of stepping down off a kerbstone as we do, they are made level with the street, the wide streets show off the buildings well. I'm sure we have almost as good buildings in Sydney but the streets are so narrow you cannot see them as well, for instance our Post Office is ever so much better, but it has not the setting. Then their Botanical Gardens are simply gorgeous, ours can't come anywhere near them, except with the view, they are simply a blaze of colour, and lovely little lakes all through, they have a water lily pond, my dears they were most beautiful, huge Japanese sacred lilies out in flower, like huge wax things, the palest pink getting deeper towards the tips, and our own lovely water lilies, reds, yellows, and white. We spent some hours in the gardens.

After leaving a water-soaked Melbourne on the afternoon of Saturday 27 February from the Williamtown breakwater, the *Ballarat* sailed on to Adelaide and Fremantle. Narrelle settled into shipboard life with her coterie of new 'best' friends. Apart from the nurses, there was Miss A. Hay who, according to Narrelle, was *a very German looking woman, but she seems nice, not a bit affected,* who went off to Government House in Adelaide to visit the governor, Lord Galway, and his wife, Lady Marie Galway, a highly intelligent and cultured woman who happened to be German. Then there was 'old Mrs Mosely' who reminded Narrelle of her mother, travelling with her daughter in law; Mrs and Miss Lawford; Miss Burgess; and Mrs Hector Robinson, wife of a naval officer, who was also pregnant and, according to Narrelle, the favourite of the boat. Mrs Robinson was, she wrote, the *most fascinating, sitting knitting socks for the soldiers, she has promised a pair to all the intending soldiers on board, and laid in a stock of wool in Melbourne.* Then there was Mr Grace, a young mining engineer, on his way to join the King Edward's Horse. In charge of the *Ballarat* was Captain Hanson, *a real old sport,* rather quiet and reserved unless he was talking about submarines and battleships. There were also a couple of doctors hoping to enlist in the medical services in London.

The *Ballarat* left Australian waters and headed out into the vast Indian Ocean. There were the usual shipboard entertainments of quoits, bingo and fancy dress parties, and time passed reasonably quickly as the *Ballarat* steamed at a maximum 13.5 knots. Narrelle's favourite pastime was to sit up on deck, balancing her writing block on her knees and writing her letters. *I generally get my pad on my knee on deck & put up an umbrella & then they think I am asleep.* But everyone had the same idea. Narrelle was frustrated by the lack of space, and intolerant of the noise made by the 50 or so children who obviously enjoyed playing outside on and around the deck. It was far better for the parents to allow their children to let off steam outside rather than keep them cooped up in the small cabins, many of which were under the waterline with no portholes. *I've never heard such a jabbering crowd in all my life, it's like being let loose in a cage of monkeys,* Narrelle mused crossly to her sister Jean.

AFTER THREE WEEKS AT SEA, THEY REACHED DURBAN IN SOUTH AFRICA. Today Durban, in KwaZulu-Natal Province, is described as the Zulu kingdom's 'seaside playground', largely famous for its cosmopolitan lifestyle and wonderful beaches. It also has the largest and busiest port in southern Africa. Built around a large natural bay, in the nineteenth century Durban (formerly known as Port Natal) was a site of conflict between the British colonial forces (who since the late eighteenth century were established further south at Cape Town), the Boers who trekked north to escape the British in the 1830s, and the Zulu nation. The British finally assumed control and annexed the area in 1844. With the discovery of gold further inland, Durban became a thriving trading centre and a launching site for gold seekers. Today Durban also has a large population of Indians, originally brought by the British as indentured labourers for the cotton and cane field industries.

Narrelle loved Durban. It was lush, tropical and exotic. Whether it was because she was glad to step onto dry land or eat a decent meal or get away from the constraints of shipboard life and the noisy children, Narrelle really enjoyed her short stay. She wrote two long letters to her mother and sister Jean describing lunch being served by Indian waiters at the upmarket Marine Hotel. *It was certainly adorable, quite tropical, you went up wide white steps on to a wider stone verandah with pillars and arches, and palms, small tables and chairs, wide doors and windows opening into sweetly clean rooms*. She also visited the zoo that was, to her amazement, so clean; had a crazy ride in a rickshaw; and visited the Museum, Art Gallery, and the fabulous recently built Renaissance-style Town Hall. During a tram ride up to the Berea Ridge, where many of the wealthy lived, Narrelle experienced the veiled hand of racism, explaining that the white people sat up the front of the tram with the black people behind them. *It's the unwritten law*, she noted cautiously. There she found superb views of the city, glimpses of the Drakensberg mountains and, far away, the ocean. Narrelle was overawed by the fabulous flame trees (or 'Flamboyant' trees) with their amazing red leaves: *they spread out from the stems just like an umbrella, soft feathery green leaves, and crimson flowers*. Then there was the night-time car trip out to Umgani, miles away.

> *My dear, it was away out, miles from the town, and perfectly beautiful, there are gardens and places there all lit up with electric lights, we wandered round for a while then as it was after 11pm we thought we had better get back to the ship, so off we went, six in each car. The first car had a puncture soon after we left, we passed them and flew on past sugar cane plantations and queer old houses covered with vines and surrounded with dense foliage, very tropical to look at, and as it was moonlight we were able to see it quite well, but we regretted it had not been daylight, but we discovered we could get out there by train if we wanted to. Just when our car, containing Dr Marsack, Captain, Mr Corbett, Miss Wellman and Miss Hobbes* [sometimes Narrelle, tongue-in-cheek, referred to herself in this formal style], *got to the P.O. we had a blow-out and had to sit on the kerbstone while a new one was put on, and in consequence only got to the boat at 12 midnight; we were glad we had the Captain with us, coaling was in full swing.*

This was Narrelle's first taste of another culture, and she found it exciting, exotic and alluring. She thoroughly enjoyed herself. But almost immediately on leaving Durban a medical crisis developed on board the *Ballarat* that would rock Narrelle to her core and bring her back to reality. A young mother and two children had embarked at Durban. One of the children, a little boy about three years old, developed an acute case of diphtheria very suddenly. Being highly contagious, the boy was placed in a cabin up on the poop deck, far away from the other passengers. A doctor performed an emergency tracheotomy to ease his breathing but it did not help. His breathing was shallow, laboured and each breath became a struggle. Narrelle and the other nurses were called on to provide a four-hour nursing roster for the sick little boy. In the early hours of the morning, during Narrelle's shift, he died. She was greatly affected by the death. *I've felt decidedly off colour all day that kiddie gave me a shock, he went off so suddenly really, heart failure, and the isolation Hospital is up on the Poop and you feel the motion of the boat very much, especially leaning over the berth,* she explained to her family in her next letter. Narrelle also described the shipboard funeral that occurred later that day.

> *... Poor little man, it was dreadfully sad, a space on the well deck was cleared and roped off, then six sailors walked along with a stretcher on which was the little body covered with the Union Jack. The Captain, Chief Officers, Dr and some of the other officers attended and most of the passengers. At the words 'we commit his body to the deep', the stretcher was raised and the little body stitched up in canvas and lead slid overboard, the boat in the meantime had been stopped, but as soon as the body was over the engines started again, one man as we passed the spot dropped a little bunch of flowers over ... it was very sad.*

Early on Friday, 26 March, the *Ballarat* reached Cape Town, a city dominated by Table Mountain towering over it. Cape Town has a much older history than Durban. The Dutch first arrived in the 1650s and established an important trading centre, warring with and eventually displacing the local Khoi people. By the 1700s, the Cape had developed into an attractive town supporting a thriving Dutch colony. It was a good half way spot for sailors and traders plying the oceans between Europe and Asia. British forces occupied Cape Town from 1795 and formally annexed it after 1814. As the British empire strengthened, the strategic benefits of the Cape came to the fore, especially with the discovery of gold in the late nineteenth century. Representative government was granted to the Cape Colony in 1853, at a similar time to that of the Australian colonies. Enmity between the Dutch, or Afrikaners, and the British simmered, finally boiling over into the South African War, or Boer War. The boundaries of the South Africa we know today were largely forged in the aftermath of that war.

By 1914 and World War I, the Cape was a vital supply and transport hub for Australian and New Zealand troops, and they all stopped off at Cape Town on their way to, and return from, war. Narrelle found Cape Town noisy, extremely busy, hot, dusty and generally disagreeable. Not even the beautiful sunrise reflected by the magnificent Table Mountain, with its deep purples against a burnt orange sun, could assuage her opinion of the place. Perhaps the novelty of travelling and tourist life had worn off, or perhaps it was the lingering images of the death of the small boy on the ship the week before. Whatever the reason, Narrelle was not impressed. To her, Cape Town was *sordid and dirty* and there was, she wrote, *a very foreign element in Cape Town, very Dutch and German.* The wharves were jammed full of troopships and supply vessels. Horses, mules and fodder were being loaded; hundreds of men in khaki uniforms were running around — all noise, dust and confusion. Many were preparing to be sent to fight in the German African colonies of German South West Africa (now Namibia) and East Africa (now broken up into Tanzania, Rwanda and Burundi). Perhaps it was for the best that the *Ballarat* only had one day in Cape Town. On 27 March, she set off for Las Palmas in the Canary Islands, and onwards towards London.

After dodging enemy submarines, the *Ballarat* and Narrelle arrived in London in mid-April 1915, to a city in the grip of an early spring and fearful of zeppelin raids. Narrelle immediately set about organising appointments and interviews. After two months at sea, she was more than ready for active service. Quite fortuitously, the situation regarding nurses had changed significantly in the two months she was on the high seas. The war in France had stalled, with fighting bogged down on the western front around Reims and Ypres. The Turkish army was causing problems for the Allies in Armenia; and on the eastern front, the Russians were faltering around the Carpathians. The great Allied gamble of a naval and military assault on the Dardanelles by French, British and Australian troops was underway.

Narrelle had a number of family friends and acquaintances to visit. Most were 'Red Crossing' for the war effort, working as VADs (Voluntary Aids) or sewing, knitting and fundraising for the British Red Cross Society or its Australian branch. Narrelle also filled in her days sightseeing. From her lodgings in Guildford Street, near Russell Square, Narrelle took in the Tate Gallery; visited the beautiful Kew Gardens, where she walked for miles in the soupy London sunshine; and enjoyed riding about in the open red double decker buses. *My dears,* she wrote, *every available square yard is used for drilling soldiers, wherever there is a spot in London large enough to allow a squad to drill and they march through the streets in hundreds.* Early May brought warm, spring-like weather. Whilst Londoners complained and wilted in the unseasonally hot weather, for Narrelle it was like a nice winter's day in Brewarrina.

Being on the spot in London made Narrelle realise the enormity and impact of the war. As she wrote:

> *... people in Australia have absolutely no idea what this war is, it's ghastly, men who have come back, invalided, all have a strained set expression on their faces, & have the most frightful nightmares, one man, when asked about his experiences was a long time before he would say anything, then he said, 'Well look Miss, its all too awful to talk about, its*

> *Hell over there, & our one desire is to try and forget it when we come away' & another man when they said 'I suppose you are longing to get better & go over again to have another shot at them' simply said 'If we are wanted we will all go back, certainly, but, our one prayer is that we may never have to go there again'.*

In one letter, written after the Gallipoli landing on 25 April, Narrelle wrote out for her family the news item published in the *Pall Mall Gazette,* written by British journalist Ashmead Bartlett, *who is supposed to be the best & more reliable man & witnessed the landing,* she gushed. Narrelle was not to know that this account was later published in Australian newspapers to much public acclaim, and provides us with the genesis of the Anzac legend. Narrelle, like all Australians at the time, loved the account, especially how it praised the actions and performance of the Australian and New Zealand troops.

Narrelle's first preference was to enlist in the Queen Alexandra's Imperial Military Nursing Service Reserve, or QAIMNSR. Rose, Elsie and Narrelle applied on 24 April, only days after arriving in London. They filled out the forms, with all their personal details, training and experience. Cheekily, on her application Narrelle stated that she was 30 years old, which was four years younger than she actually was. This placed her mid-range in the age quota, which may have been her motivation. She also stated that she was 'twice charge nurse of enteric wards for six months at a time', something she may or may not have actually done.

The QAIMNS was the main British military nursing service whose history dated back to Florence Nightingale and the Crimean War. From 1866, civilian nurses were appointed to military hospitals. Women were gradually accepted, albeit grudgingly, into the army nursing service with the formation of Princess Christian's Army Nursing Reserve in 1881. But it was really during the Boer War that female military nursing became firmly established. The appalling medical casualties suffered during that conflict by the British troops were largely attributed to disease and neglect rather than direct battle injuries. Several Royal Commissions were established afterwards to investigate various aspects of the war. As part of a series of reforms of the British military, the Queen Alexandra's Imperial Military Nursing Service or QAIMNS was established in March 1902. Named after Queen Alexandra, wife of King Edward VII, the QAIMNS enjoyed royal patronage. Queen Alexandra designed the QAIMNS badge as a cross, with the Danish royal arms (her father was the King of Denmark), surrounded by an Imperial Crown, with the letter 'A' within a circle, surrounded by an oval band bearing the inscription QAIMNS. The motto of the QAIMNS was *sub cruce candida*, translated as 'Under the White Cross'. The uniform was a striking grey and scarlet.

Attached to the British army and working closely with its medical arm, the Royal Army Medical Corps (RAMC), the QAIMNS were divided into two sections, the regulars and the reserves. There were about 300 regulars in 1914 but for some reason the reserves were not popular. On the other hand, the Territorial Force Nursing Service (or the 'Terriers' as they were fondly nicknamed), a nursing reserve formed in 1908 as part of the new Territorial Reserves Forces Act, appealed to many young nurses and, on the outbreak of war in September 1914, had about 2000 nurses available for war service.

It is said that timing is everything, and Narrelle and her nursing friends from the *Ballarat* certainly arrived in London at the right time. Whilst there was always a demand for properly trained and experienced nurses throughout the war, the British authorities were overwhelmed by the unexpected chaos of the Gallipoli campaign and the huge medical and logistical problems that resulted from the first weeks of horrendous fighting on the Turkish peninsula. Additional nurses were urgently required to staff the hospital ships, hospitals and convalescent facilities that were hastily established in Egypt, Lemnos and Malta.

After anxiously waiting two weeks for a response to her application,

Narrelle enlisted the help of Dr W.P. Norris, from the Australian Commonwealth Medical Bureau in London, in her quest for an interview with the matron-in-chief of the QAIMNS, Miss Ethel Becher. Narrelle wanted some indication of whether the QAIMNS would be interested in her application, or whether she should take up Miss Birt's original offer to work at the Red Cross Hospital at Huntingdon. Through Narrelle's correspondence we can glimpse the chaos and confusion within the ranks of the British medical establishment. On 5 May, Narrelle described what happened in a letter home.

> *On Monday, first thing, I trotted around to Dr Norris he was very charming as usual, & gave me a letter to take to the War Office myself, it is some distance from Victoria Street nearly up to Charing X past Westminster, a huge grey block. Dr Norris had told me what to do, fortunately, for I assure you its a great business getting inside the War Office these times, met one Bobbie* [policeman] *at the first door, he passed me on to a 2nd who passed me into a room filled with men & soldiers, all busy filling in papers, an attendant there gave me a pink paper with questions to fill in … this was passed on to a man in uniform, who read it through then yelled, 'Is Sister Hobbes present' — a smile went round all the room, & I shouted back, over the heads of dozens of them 'Yes' then a Boy Scout was called & again the voice called 'Sister Hobbes, & Sergeant–something–follow the boy' & we followed. The Ser — grinned & saluted me, we seemed to walk for miles through wide echoing halls & up lifts, Sister Hobbes wishing that Kitchener & some of the other great men would pass along. At last we came to a standstill before another policeman, who asked us our business & I was shown into a waiting room filled once more with men, nice clean looking English boys, &, I am sure from their brown leanness, some Australian boys, there to volunteer. Presently a plump little woman came trotting along & beckoned me out, & asked what I wanted, I gave her my letter from Dr Norris & said I wanted to see if it would make any difference to my getting a permanent military appointment if I went up there* [to Huntingdon with Miss Birt], *or if it*

would be better to remain in London in case I was accepted & wanted. She trotted off again & presently came back & said, in rather an offhand way, 'Miss Beecher [Becher] *says take it by all means there is no reason whatever why you should not'.*

Well, they say persistence pays off for, after more problems with mistaken identity, Matron Becher herself came out to speak with the young Australian nurse.

Presently a rather sweet faced nurse in the grey army service uniform with red collar & tabs, came along & beckoned me out, said she was very sorry the mistake had been made, she was very busy & had just glanced at the name, & then reading it again had found the initial different & was my name Nar-rel-lie Hobbes, & I hadn't a e in it', so I put her on the right track, & she said 'Well I think you might as well go up to Miss Birt & relieve her, but write & let me know a few days before you are to leave Huntingdon, & I will know you are free. Your papers are in our hands but have not all been gone through yet, but be sure & let me know before you leave Huntingdon'.

Narrelle never made it to Huntingdon. To her absolute delight, she was accepted by the War Office into the QAIMNS Reserve before she could make the arrangements. The need for experienced nurses was so great that no references were required, just the written reports from her matron back in Australia, which she had already submitted with her application. The following day Narrelle received a reply-paid cable: *Would you go Malta or Egypt on short notice.* Jumping for joy, Narrelle shouted with delight, and wired back immediately, *Yes either place where ordered.* Her fate was sealed. Narrelle was thrilled that Rose and Elsie were also accepted into the QAIMNSR. They were then informed that all three would be embarking for Malta in three days. Just enough time to get their military uniforms, nurses' kit, and belongings organised. So, *off we flew & got to Shoolbreeds (Shortbread) I call him, it's less German. We measured & saw our clothing ... Nurses going to Malta or Egypt must have hats instead of bonnets large brimmed grey straw with a little band of that stiff sort of Petersham ribbon with red, white & blue stripes running round the crown & a weird little bow at the side. They are all the same size with a bit of velvet inside, which if you have a small head you draw up — if a large head you cut it out — as R. Kirkaldie has red hair & bright & bright colour if you can imagine what the red of the uniform looks like against it poor dear, fortunately that is only the outside. We are not allowed to take 1 article of private clothing, we do not wear stiff collars being 'Malta'. It was very funny in Shortbreads, in the outfit room you were asked are you a 'Malta' or 'Egypt' Sister? After fixing up our uniforms etc in the regular outfit you are allowed 8 aprons, 3 dresses (indoor) — grey zepher, so I thank my stars I had some extra for I would be always be running out of them, why that meant only 4 aprons a week.*

Within days, Narrelle, Rose and Elsie were aboard the *Mongolia*, steaming towards Gibraltar, en route to Malta in the Mediterranean, with a contingent of nurses, other medical staff and medical provisions. Despite Narrelle's initial frustration at the apparent slowness of the British medical establishment, it had, in fact, only taken one month from her arrival in London to her departure as a QAIMNS nurse. The pay and conditions were not great — indeed it was less than what she received in Australia — but as she wrote to her family, *there is little to spend your money on when you're on 'Active Service'*. Her salary, she informed her family, was £50 per annum as a nursing sister with an annual increment of £5 to a maximum of £65. Wages for a matron were £75 reaching a maximum of £150 per annum. There was also a gratuity on leaving the QAIMNS, which, unlike the Australian system, was graded according to rank. An annual clothing and cloak allowance, plus outfit allowance when proceeding on active service, was also included.

In a letter to the Australasian Trained Nurses' Association (ATNA), which was later published in their journal, Narrelle wrote encouraging

Australian nurses, saying that they would be *practically sure of an appointment somewhere* if they came over. She also described the nursing contingent with her on the *Mongolia*.

There are 40 nurses on board — 19 Canadians, 10 Imperial, and 10 Red Cross Nurses, and at meals it is really rather pretty. The Canadians all wear light blue frocks, white aprons and caps, and sit at one end of the table; then we ten military nurses with our grey frocks, little grey capes with scarlet edges, and white caps and cuffs, and little soft white turn-over collars; then the British Red Cross Nurses [VAs] *in the dark blue frocks, white aprons and caps. We have one long table reserved for the nurses, and we just fill it.*

The *Mongolia* crossed the Bay of Biscay where the ship was chased by a German submarine, which they eluded by zigzagging through the water. The submarine was also, perhaps, outbluffed by the gun, mounted menacingly on the ship's deck. The rough seas and fast pace of the boat may have advantaged the *Mongolia* but created havoc for its passengers who were all violently seasick. There was a short stop at Gibraltar, whose harbour was packed with at least nine British warships, for last minute stores and supplies, and to remove the torpedo nets and guns. Narrelle's last letter before reaching Malta was written to her sister Grace on 22 May as they steamed towards their destination. She was tentative, uncertain and nervous.

My dearest old Grace,

Only a scrawl this time, I'm just trying to write a few lines to <u>all</u>, in case we have not time for writing when once we get to Malta, as I am sure we will not, as they have 8,000 wounded, or had when we heard last, and the day we were at Gibraltar we heard they were overflowing 500 to Gib, they were expected that day poor souls, it's ghastly really. We expect to be sent on to the Dardanelles later on as they are forming a *base Hospital there, and will want Nurses* ... [This never happened. No hospitals were ever established on Gallipoli, so no nurses were ever stationed on the peninsula].

Malta is in sight and we are all suffering from stage fright, wondering what we are in for, in the way of people to live with and work for. You simply don't know the horror of it, going to perfectly strange people in a strange land with strange methods, every nurse hates it, even in our own country it's beastly, and the English nurses are noted for their treatment of Australian nurses. They don't like us, never have and never will, they are jealous, as we are really better trained than they are, and have a higher standard, you only have to come over here and see them to know that, however, we are all agreed that we will meet them half way and be quite nice to all, and ready to accept their methods, it's too much to think that we might be able to keep together, where-ever we go.
Must stop & try & write Kit & Josie a few lines.

Oceans of love to all from Narrie.

And so to Malta, active service and war.

P&O.S.N.Co.
S.S. Mongolia
May 22nd

My dearest old Grace,

Only a scrawl this time, I'm just trying to write a few lines to all, in case we have not time for writing when once we get to Malta, as I am sure we will not, as they have 8'000 wounded, or had when we heard last, & the day we were at Gibraltar we heard they were overflowing 500 to Gib, they were expected that day poor souls, its ghastly really, we expect to be sent on to the Dardanelles later on as they are forming a base Hospital there.

The first and last page of Narrelle's letter to sister Grace Weston, written on her way to Malta, 22 May 1915. (*Hobbes Collection*) their methods, its too much to think that we might be able to keep together, where-ever we go.

Must stop & try & write Kit & Josie a few lines.

Oceans of love to all from

Narrie.

Do write often dear, even if there is no news, fancy its 3 weeks on Monday since we had any Australian mail, Monday before last there was no mail in, then we had to leave the day before it arrived & we've been just a week at sea, & it will be another week or fortnight before we get it, awful.

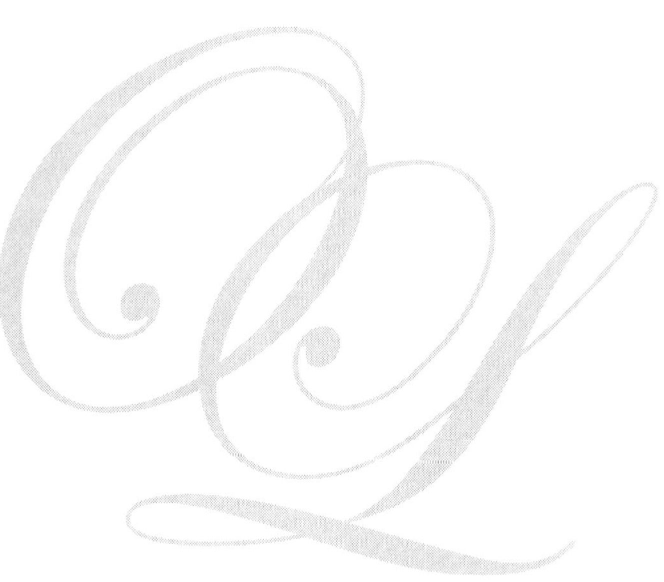

Malta

Chapter 3

'Always Somebody's Boy'

A tiny archipelago, Malta is situated at the crossroads of the Mediterranean Sea, 60 miles (96 kilometres) south of Sicily, east of ancient Carthage, now modern day Tunis, and about 125 miles (200 kilometres) north of Tripoli at the top of the African continent. Its three largest islands — Gozo, Comino and Malta — are inhabited but have no fresh water, limited arable land, and a largely rocky limestone terrain. Malta's value has always been its strategic geographic position. The Maltese people have traditionally survived on military and later naval activities, from the Knight Crusaders to the British Forces. Today, fishing and tourism keeps Malta's economy operating; its pleasant Mediterranean climate of mild, wet winters and dry, hot summers are particularly enticing for British and Northern European visitors. There are spectacular ruins ranging from pre-Roman sites to Crusader forts for tourists to clamber over and explore. The medieval town of Medina, once the capital, with its cobbled streets and cathedral, sits nestled in the middle of the island of Malta, offering magnificent views of the island, and the sparkling turquoise blue of the Mediterranean.

Because of its geographical position, Malta has been fought over and influenced by different empires for over a thousand years. From the Phoenicians and Carthaginians, to the Greeks, Romans and Islamic Sultans, Malta has been considered a prized possession. In 1530,

Charles V allowed the Knights of St John, more famously known as the Knights of Malta, to settle there. Surviving the great siege of Malta in 1565 against the Ottoman Turks, they built fortresses, harbours, towns, churches, and hospitals. The Knights were also responsible for building the town of Valletta, now the capital of Malta, nestled around one of the finest harbours in Europe. And the Knights' hospital at Valletta soon became renowned as one of the world's best. Napoleon briefly held Malta from 1798 until the British formally annexed the island in 1814 at the end of the Napoleonic Wars.

Through the decades of the nineteenth century as Britain became a premier naval power, Malta, with its deep natural harbours and heavy fortifications was built up as a significant and strategic naval base. The British installed a governor and built warehouses, a dock for shipbuilding, and other essential infrastructure to support both mercantile and military interests in the Mediterranean. During the Crimean War of 1854–56, Malta became an important medical base for the treatment of wounded soldiers. Whilst the war was a turning point for the development of women and nursing through the exploits of Florence Nightingale and others, it also gave Malta a new role, and a new nickname, as the 'Nurse of the Mediterranean'. In the aftermath of the Crimean War, Royal Commissions were held to improve and revamp the military medical facilities. New hospitals were built on both Malta and Gozo. At the outbreak of World War I, there were four hospitals on Malta. The largest was the Valletta Military Hospital with 232 beds, and quarters for members of the RAMC stationed on the island. Then there was the Cottonera Hospital with about 150 beds; the Forrest Hospital, which largely used tents and was for infectious diseases; and the convalescent hospital, Citta Vecchia Sanitarium.

By February 1915, with the assault on the Dardanelles in the final planning stages, it became clear that the medical facilities currently operating in Egypt would not be sufficient in an emergency. Expanding the medical facilities on Malta was an obvious solution. Malta was halfway between the Gallipoli peninsula and Gibraltar. Hospital ships could steam

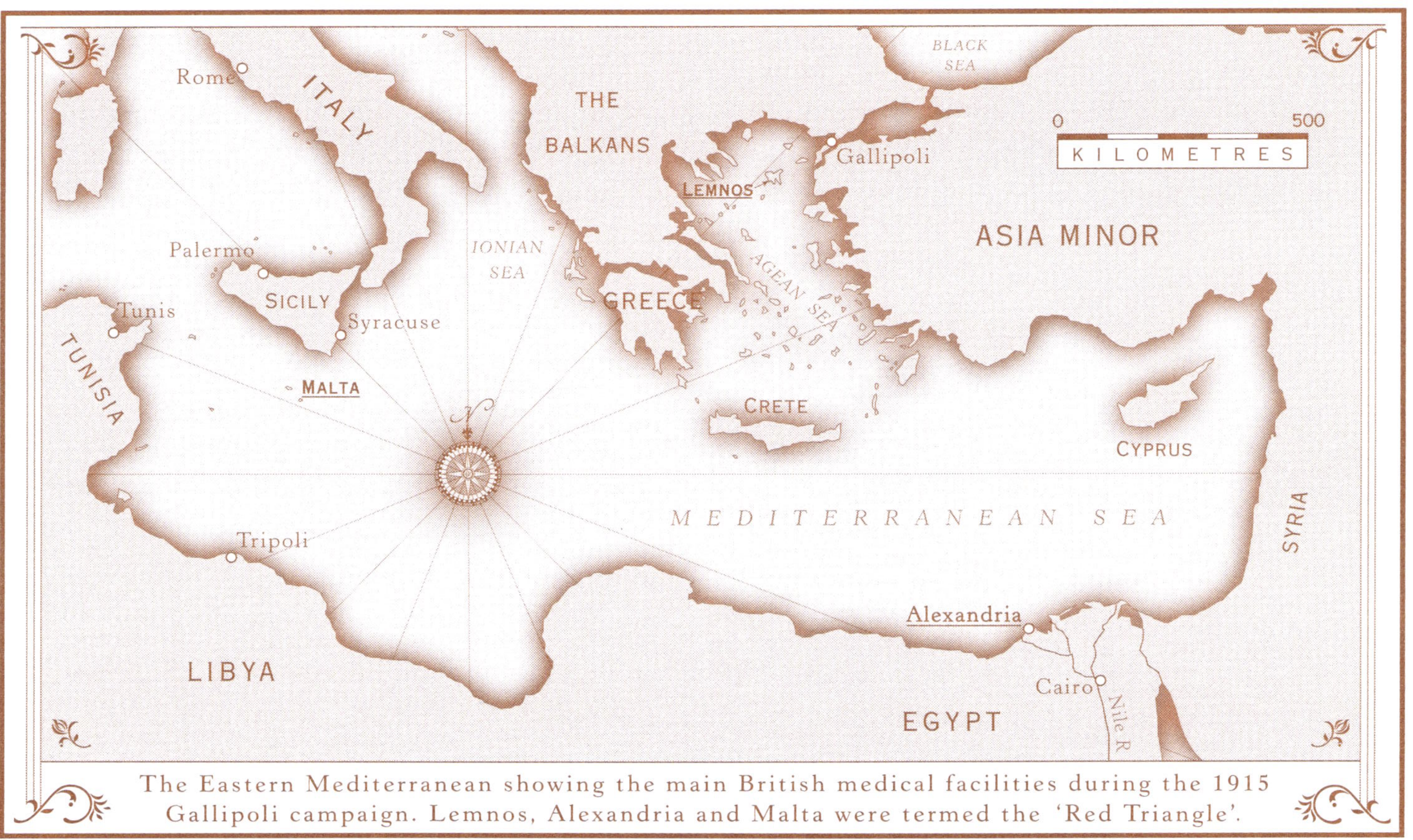

The Eastern Mediterranean showing the main British medical facilities during the 1915 Gallipoli campaign. Lemnos, Alexandria and Malta were termed the 'Red Triangle'.

there within days. The development of Malta as a fully operational medical facility would also take the pressure off British hospitals in Egypt. The red triangle of British medical facilities for the Gallipoli campaign became Lemnos (an island off the coast of Greece), Alexandria in Egypt, and Malta. It was 650 miles (1040 kilometres) from Lemnos to Alexandria and a further 820 miles (1312 kilometres) from Alexandria to Malta. Lemnos to Malta direct was 850 miles (1360 kilometres).

NARRELLE HOBBES ARRIVED IN MALTA AS PART OF THE LARGE MEDICAL response by British authorities to cope with the carnage on Gallipoli in the spring of 1915. Hundreds of doctors, orderlies, nurses, medical equipment and supplies were rushed to Malta to assist with the casualties from the fighting. During May alone, over 200 nurses, 82 medical officers and 798 RAMC orderlies arrived. By September, there were over 2500 medical staff on the island.

The first boatload of wounded and sick men from Gallipoli, about 600 patients in all, turned up at Malta on 4 May, three weeks before Narrelle's arrival. Despite his best preparations, Lord Methuen, governor and commander-in-chief in Malta, and his skeleton medical staff were overwhelmed by the numbers of wounded, and by their horrendous condition. The men were crammed onto the ship, lying cheek by jowl on a deck open to the elements, with wounds festering in the spring heat and held together with dirty bandages unchanged since leaving Gallipoli days earlier. It was simply appalling. Inadequate staff to assist the patients only exacerbated the situation. To make matters worse, it took hours to offload the men from the ship to barges, which then ferried them to shore. After medical inspections, delayed again by a lack of staff, the patients were eventually categorised into severe, urgent, and non-urgent cases, and despatched to the appropriate hospital.

And this was not a one-off. The hospital ships just kept on coming. By the end of May, just after Narrelle arrived, there were over 4000 casualties on the island. Narrelle and her colleagues were thrown into the deep end. No wonder she had 'stage fright' and was nervous. She had had almost no training whatsoever for military nursing. She had never dealt with gunshot, bayonet or shell wounds. Nor had she seen festering, mangled, gangrenous flesh wounds hastily treated. The reality of war and its consequences confronted her first hand. Although Narrelle did not know it yet, she was taking part in what would become 'Australia's baptism of fire', an event that would help shape and define a nation. And whilst we rarely hear their voices or tell their stories, Narrelle, and the hundreds of Australian nurses like her in the AANS, the QAIMNS, and the Red Cross were part of the story that we now know as Gallipoli.

On arrival in Malta, there was no time to reflect and barely any time to write home to her family about what she was doing. Narrelle was posted to the Valletta Military Hospital, originally built by the Knights of Malta, under Matron Brown, a veteran from the Boer War. This hospital had been extended, and housed the ward famous for its size that contained over 200 beds. As it was closest to the wharves where the ships docked, Valletta Hospital generally handled the most serious medical and surgical cases. In the shady courtyard adjacent to the hospital, weekly evening concerts were held to entertain the patients. Narrelle described the hospital in a letter home.

> *It's a part of two sides, the two arches being the stairways to the wards up and down, the walls are mostly covered with odd creepers, plumbago trained right up, & a red flower & a yellow feathery thing. The yard is paved with huge old stones & the building is of huge stones, walls nearly 3 feet through, built about 1520 or thereabouts. In the centre of the compound is an old, old fountain, said fountain now dry & filled with earth & flowers growing in it. Then at one end just opposite my wards, they rigged a stage with flags etc all round, & commandeered all the chairs they could find. I wish you could have seen the collection of patients, they had bandages on every portion of their anatomy, some had crutches, some just*

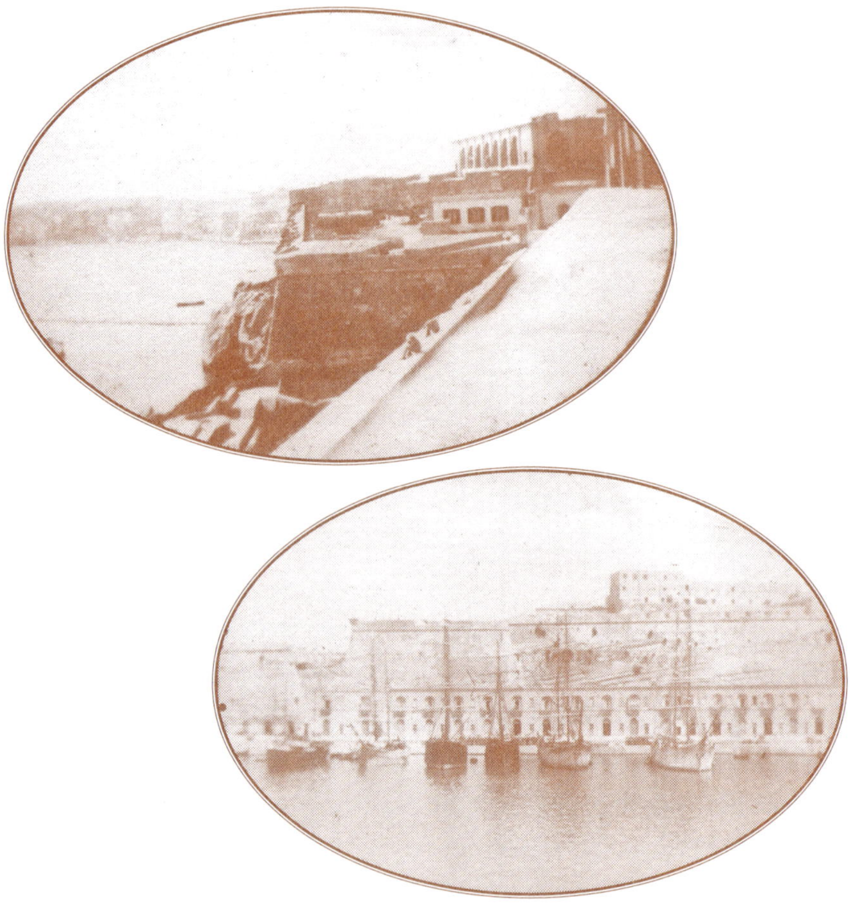

Photographs of Valletta, Malta, taken by Narrelle and sent back to her family in Australia, 1915. (*Hobbes Collection*)

> *walked, but all came who could, then there were men in uniform wherever you looked … it was hard to believe we were only a few days off such ghastly sights. They* [the concerts] *always start about 7.30 & go till 9 pm.*

During the war over twenty hospitals with more than 7000 beds were established on Malta. These included hospitals for slightly wounded men, surgical hospitals, and infectious diseases hospitals, including venereal disease. There were vast tent hospitals, convalescent homes and rest camps, such as the Ghain Tuffieha Camp, with its cool breezes and perfect bathing conditions on the western side of the island about 10 miles (16 kilometres) from Valletta, which could accommodate upwards of 3000 men. The British Red Cross Society established a hospital at Hamrun in the basement of the technical school in June 1915, later taken over by the military. The hospitals were administered directly from Malta, not the War Office in London, with medical supplies, equipment and personnel being sent from Britain when requested. Nursing staff was billeted at the Cammerata, which had been the quarters for married soldiers, and was directly opposite the main Valletta Hospital. In all, over 2500 officers and 55,400 soldiers were evacuated to Malta and treated in its hospitals during the eight months of the Gallipoli campaign. Many thousands who needed ongoing hospitalisation were transferred to England whilst others ready again for active service were sent back to Egypt or direct to the peninsula.

On 20 June, almost one month after Narrelle arrived in Malta, on a rare quiet afternoon off duty, she wrote to her family. She had much to say about her work and routine, and the types of patients she was caring for. Through Narrelle's descriptions, we get a good idea of what conditions were like for nurses, and how she coped with the stress of active service. Most of all, Narrelle was thrilled to be nursing Australians and New Zealanders, her favourite patients. She also mentioned a story about a man with a donkey, revealing just how quickly the Simpson account became part of the folklore of Gallipoli.

Dearest People,

There is really nothing to write about this week, there is nothing but work to discuss. We've been very busy till the last 48 hours, & now we are expecting in 100 cot cases (meaning in the language of the military 'bad cases') this afternoon, and are just lying in wait for the call to the wards. Do you know I absolutely cannot cast my mind back to my last letter & think of what has gone on in the meantime, I only know I get up at 6.30, breakfast at 7 am, on duty 7.30, lunch either 12.30 or 1 o'clock, it all depends what time we are supposed to go off, when we can we take it in turns about going off from 1 to 4.30 or from 4.30 for the rest of the day, but its so desperately hot here that your one desire is to get your clothes off & throw yourself on the bed till it's time to go on again. All the shops close from 1 to 3 pm in the summer.

We are sending every patient who is able to travel to England tomorrow, my nice New Z and Australian boys are off with them, I shall miss them very much … They have been longing to go to England so yesterday the Colonel came round with papers to fill in getting the names of all the men who could go, I handed in two of them I knew could go … they go off to-morrow morning, till fit for active service again. Poor men, I hate to think of them going back again. You know it's only when you get tales first hand like we do here, from the men who have been right through it that you begin to realise the least little bit what it is like.

I must tell you the story of a poor R.A.M.C. man, that somehow made me think of Mr Andrews [her friend from Brewarrina]. *This man got hold of a donkey and used to go backwards & forwards to the firing line, & putting the wounded on the donkey would convey him to the 1st aid place. For a fortnight he was known all along the line as the man with the donkey, &, as he passed the men would cheer him, but one day he never passed, & then they found him. He & the donkey were dead.*

My dears, the things these boys tell us, one boy said to me one day when I was washing him 'Sister there is one thing I am thankful to be away from the trenches for & that is to get away from the insects — lice — they crawled all over you, from head to foot', and I can quite believe it. We were once told we were not to touch a man when the wounded arrived till the orderlies had washed & cleaned them, but you've got to or you would never get done.

A Hospital ship from the Dardanelles came in the day before yesterday, but the men were beautifully clean & well looked after, as they had 9 or 10 sisters on board which makes all the difference. When they just come over in a transport they arrive in a filthy condition poor dears, they are simply crowded on, lie on deck or stretchers or anything, with about two or three sisters & two doctors for hundreds of men, & they simply can't look after them. Consequently they are fearfully septic & limbs have to be amputated that might have been saved, it's appalling the number of amputations that have to be done.

… My dears, you say you had your first real touch of the war when the casualty list came out, that's nothing, I thought that too, when I first read the lists, but it's only when you see them brought in stretcher after stretcher in that endless procession and wonder if, when you see the next man's face, if you will see one of your own friends, dear heaven, it's awful, & every man or boy … is 'somebody's boy'. There are times when we wonder if we can keep right along at it, but not often, for I for one will never give it up till we are not needed.

The working conditions for Narrelle and the medical staff were daunting, to say the least. The Maltese summer was well underway and this made the situation even more trying. Narrelle mentioned the dreaded sirocco, that dry, hot wind from North Africa, which brought with it a fine, soft, powdery dust. It covered everything in a white powder — the houses, the streets, the shop awnings — and made living conditions trying in the extreme. Despite living in western New South Wales, where hot summers with temperatures over 100 degrees Fahrenheit (38 degrees Celsius) were commonplace, Narrelle found acclimatising to the Maltese summer very challenging.

The heat of Malta is disgusting, very moist, the perspiration just pours off you, & then the Sirocco is rotten, Sydney weather in the middle of summer on a moist day is delightful compared with this. Now, for instance to-day, apparently just to look outside there is a clear blue sky & bright sun shining, & as long as you don't move everything is delightful, move & the sweat runs off you, hot & sticky, & you ache in every joint as though you were just getting flu, & all your boots are two sizes too small. I have a half day, came off after lunch & meant to write reams all round, but was so tired when I got to my room, I thought I would have a rest first, got undressed & lay on my bed, & went sound asleep, but when I wakened I absolutely could not move I was aching all over. At last after about an hour I simply made myself get up & went & stood in a hip bath & poured a few jugs of water over myself for a shower bath, after which I put on a dress & singlet & went down for some afternoon tea as I found I had no paraffin in my lamp (if you ask for kerosene here they don't know what you mean). I must try & get some, but now I'm trying to get some letters written I promised to write for my poor old helpless patients, they think so much of any little thing like that.

DEALING WITH THE CASUALTIES FIRST HAND HELPED NARRELLE understand what the men were going through on the Dardanelles. She saw the wounds of her patients and tried to heal them; she witnessed their pain and suffering and tried to soothe them; she talked and listened to them in order to console them. She also scoured the casualty lists for men that she knew, and then tried to find them.

I see poor Wilfred Hartridge has been wounded, I must go … and see if he is on the Island. He is the nice youngster from the Brewarrina Bush Brothers …

Narrelle did find Wilfred and managed to spend some time with him. He had received a gunshot wound to the hand and was also suffering from bronchitis, presumably left over from the pneumonia he contracted en route to Egypt from Australia. Wilfred recovered from his wounds and chest complaints, and returned to the peninsula. A month later the 21 year old was dead. It is not known exactly when he died but he took part in the battle for Lone Pine. As a member of the 3rd Battalion of the Australian Infantry, he died sometime between 7 and 12 August 1915. No-one knows for sure. The dead were left in the hot summer heat. It was impossible to retrieve their bodies. According to Charles Bean, the official Australian war correspondent and later historian, the losses of the 3rd Battalion (which went into the battle with 23 officers and 736 soldiers) was 21 officers and 490 soldiers.

> *The boys tell such ghastly tales of how men have lain outside the trenches for hours & no one could get to them — they have jumped up on the trench suddenly & hurled their water bottles to the man outside & couldn't get high enough to shoot — & end everything for the poor souls, oh & tales that make ones blood turn to water — almost — how they stand it the way they do I do not know, but it makes me feel that you can't do enough for them.*

Lone Pine was a battle intended to divert the enemy's attention from the main game at the British held positions of Sari Bair further down the peninsula. It was a complete and utter disaster from the Australian point of view. Hartridge was but one of 2197 Australian men and 80 officers killed during three days of fierce, often hand-to-hand combat. The Turks suffered enormous casualties too. It was a blood bath all round, for almost no gain whatsoever. On hearing the news of Wilfred's death, Narrelle confided in a letter of 5 October ... *poor Wilfred H — he was such a favourite — hope it was instantaneous* ... His personal effects, including a prayer book, stone curios, cards and a handkerchief, letters and photographs, were sent home to his mother in England.

The reality of war continued to impact directly on Narrelle's world. She noted that Geoff Yeomans, another young man from Brewarrina, was injured with shrapnel wounds to his left arm in late May. Yeomans, from the AIF's 1st Battalion, recovered and returned to Gallipoli on 12 July. Within a year he, too, was dead, killed in action in France.

Promoted to lieutenant, Yeomans died on 22 July 1916 at the start of the battle of Pozières Ridge on the Somme. Narrelle also met up with the other Brewarrina Bush Brother, 28-year-old Leonard (Leo) Andrews, on Malta. Andrews, an Englishman from Stoke Newington, and a clerk in Holy Orders had enlisted as a private in the 1st Field Ambulance Reinforcements, and embarked from Australia on 11 February 1915, only days before Narrelle. She knew he was on Gallipoli, but believed the chances of meeting up were slim. However, Andrews had been evacuated to Mudros with dysentery, and Narrelle described her complete surprise and delight when one day she *had been feeling beastly bluey all the morning — I heard someone walking along the road in front of our tent & looked up — saw a uniform that I knew didn't belong to our Camp so bent down to see who it was & at the same time the man outside ducked to see who was inside — I nearly fell off my perch in my excitement — it was Mr Andrews with an absolutely colossal grin on his ugly old face — he was supposed to be in Lemnos left Alex—for there but in the boat came on here instead & he got my address from poor Wilfred* [Hartridge] *just a few days before he left the Peninsula sick … Mr Andrews & Gilbert* [Anschau, Narrelle's cousin] *who had dugouts besides each other & told them about my letter & where I was — that's how they both knew. Mr Andrews saw Holt* [Hardy] *one day looking very fit — had helped to carry Geoff Yeomans down to Anzac Cove when Geoff was wounded — I also had a letter from Holt the other day — he said Tonie* [Hordern] *& Geoff were both back in again* [on Gallipoli] *after their trip to Malta.*

Another jackaroo from 'Weilmoringle' and a friend of Narrelle's, Holt Hardy, enlisted in the 6th Australian Light Horse in September 1914. He was a typical Anzac — almost 6 feet tall, with a long angular face, grey eyes, brown hair, and a dark complexion. Holt featured regularly in her letters, and they corresponded frequently throughout the war. Aged 21, he landed on Anzac Cove on 20 May 1915, and managed to stay clear of both injury and disease for the next seven months, an amazing feat. Tonie Hordern was another of the 'Weilmoringle' jackaroos who, after a chance meeting with Narrelle on Malta, kept in touch throughout the war. From Kirribilli in Sydney, and part of the well-known Sydney retail family of Anthony Horderns, Tonie attended Sydney Grammar School. On leaving school he went jackarooing at 'Weilmoringle'. Of average height, with a dark complexion, brown eyes, black hair, and a slight build, he enlisted in the 1st Australian Light Horse on the 25 August 1914, in the first weeks of the war. As Narrelle wrote in great detail:

> *I had a cable from Mr Hordern on Wed. saying Tonie was wounded, in Malta. Would I find out if it was dangerous, & would he come over. Well I set to work to try and find him. I got my ward Sgt. to try & get on to the Castille* [headquarters] *to find where he was, it was Thursday afternoon before I could find him, so I got an afternoon pass & made for Pembroke Convalescent Camp* [later called St Paul's Camp Hospital, built with 34 huts despatched from England], *where the boy had been sent. It takes nearly an hour to get there in a Carrozzin* [a horsedrawn taxi carrying up to four people], *& then we (I took another sister along with me) had to wander around through the most awful white dust, in & out of tents till we found the orderly tent. Hot? Well give me Brewarrina with a 116 temp any day than Pembroke camp in summer. One of the men set off to find Tonie while another brought us camp seats, & we waited. It had not struck me he would be out there, so I did not take an umbrella, fortunately Sister Ramsay had, then after a while Tonie came along & I wanted to hug him. What a dear youngster he is, but he is the colour of an Arab, & so thin, & looked so tall in his shorts, you know most of the Australians have cut their pants short, over their knees, & the putties only come to the knee. Well they look the quaintest, dirtiest souls you could imagine, some of their poor uniforms are* <u>*decidedly*</u> *the worse for wear, & if you could see some of the clothes they go off to London in, with anything in the way of head gear they can get, but quite happy. But to continue about Tonie, he came along wondering, I think, who on earth could want him, for he looked at me in a puzzled way till I told him who I was, then he grasped my hand, and nearly broke the bones.*
>
> *I thought he was not looking at all well, and felt pretty mad to think he had been sent out there, & was intensely sorry he had not been sent to*

Valletta Hospital instead of the Hospital he did go to. I feel sure he was not really fit to be sent out there, where there are no Sisters, & the men just look after themselves, & they have to scramble for their meals, there are so many of them 1,110. I asked Tonie if he got good food, he said 'Oh yes, but I haven't felt inclined for food for a few days'. Well it worried me some, to think of that boy out there and not feeling well or eating, & none to look after them, so uncared for somehow, and the heat & dust. The shops were all shut by the time we got in to town, so next day I got a morning pass & rooted round & got him some bovril & tins of unsweetened milk, biscuits, chocolate & coffee, and got my VAD girl to drop them at the orderly tent as she went past the camp next day. She & her Aunt were taking some of my patients out in a car, and were passing Pembroke. [The large influx of medical staff and patients placed pressure on resources, as they had to be fed and watered. Only fresh vegetables and fruit were supplied from Malta itself. The rest of the food requirements, such as chickens and eggs, were shipped in from Italy, Egypt and Tunis.]

I've not seen or heard anything of Tonie since, & am wondering if he has been sent back to Egypt, some went back the other day. Heavens I wish I had a few hundred £s that are being gathered in Australia, just to get little comforts & things for the patients things no-one thinks of sending, just little things in their way. Now <u>*toothbrushes,*</u> *to get a toothbrush you have to give the Name, Rank, regiment, number, service, age, and any other old thing you can rake up, & then sign it & get the patient to sign it, send it down by an orderly to the ordinance store & then as likely as not they will send back & tell you that you've not put the number of the bed, or the ward or some other damn thing, & then finally it will go down again only to find they are out of them or some other old thing, & you wonder where the millions of £s are going to that Australia alone is sending, especially when you read some of the letters in the papers.*

Also embarking with Tonie on the HMAT *Star of Victoria* on 20 October 1914, was his close school friend Frederick Alexander (always called Alex) Guthrie. Tonie and Alex were typical of thousands of young

Australian men who enlisted in the first heady months of war. Almost 21 years old on enlistment, Alex had been a senior cadet at Sydney Grammar. He was 5 foot 10 inches tall, with brown hair, grey eyes and a fair complexion. Alex and Tonie managed to stay together for three years. They fought on Gallipoli, and whilst Tonie was sent to Malta for a gunshot wound to his head and arm on 29 June, Alex was later hospitalised for enteritis on Mudros in August 1915 (Narrelle refers to this in a letter). After the evacuation of the peninsula, Alex and Tonie returned to Egypt where they continued with the Light Horse, both being promoted to lieutenant in December 1916. Almost a year later, on 3 November 1917, Alex Guthrie was killed in action as part of the Australian attack at Tel Khuweilfeh, Beersheeba. He was buried in the west corner of Gum Tree Grove, Beersheeba, the following day.

His bereaved mother, Ada, and father, Frederick Guthrie, who worked at the Department of Agriculture in Sydney, received a wooden case of their son's possessions in February 1918. Over eighteen months later, in September 1919, a further small package arrived from the Middle East. It contained the following: one sheepskin vest, one muffler, one balaclava, one wooden spoon, quantity of rifle parts, one leather pouch, one pack cards, one dictionary, one pair mittens, three pairs socks, military notes, photos and one pair spur leathers. The last vestiges of their son's life had been returned to them. Whilst this would not assuage the sorrow of their bereavement, at least they had concrete information about his death, and his meagre possessions. Alex Guthrie also has a Commonwealth War Grave headstone where he was officially commemorated. Forty-five miles (72 kilometres) south-west of Jerusalem, nestled in the beautiful Beersheeba War Cemetery, surrounded by gum trees, palms and colourful flowers, is the final resting place for this young Australian. Unfortunately this was not the case for many other grieving Australian families. Over two thirds of Australians killed in World War I, about 40,000 men, have no known grave as their bodies were either never found or were unrecognisable, and therefore unidentifiable.

Narrelle did not embellish her letters, and when it came to her work, she rarely told it like it was. She witnessed terrible sights — death, men with horrendous wounds, and the ravages of diseases such as typhoid, dysentery, and the effects of louse infestations. She suffered from nightmares revolving around bandaging and dressing wounds of soldiers from which she often woke bathed in sweat. As she was working in the specialist ward in Valletta Hospital, she received the worst cases and saw indescribable things, but she rarely mentioned them in any detail in her letters home. Only when writing to her nursing friend, Smithie, did she go into any details. Whether Narrelle was holding back because she did not want to worry her family (much like the soldiers) or whether she was worried about the censor is unclear. Perhaps she knew and expected that all her family would read the letters, younger members and children included, and so she wrote them for a 'family audience'. Whatever the reason, Narrelle's letters reveal a level of restraint and self-censorship when describing her work, and the effects of her work. 'Worth', one of her first patients, and one of her favourites, is an example of this stoic attitude. In a letter home, she wrote how.

I want you to meet two of my boys when they go back to Australia, especially Worth, he is the cutest soul possible. I had him for an hour one evening trying to pick a flower up off his bed and carry it to his nose, and he was so excited when he did it, that he nearly wept, and amused himself for ages doing it over and over again, it was most pathetic. His people are not well off, they have something to do with the water works at Wagga, I'd get you to look after him when he gets to Sydney, but he would be too heavy a case, and would want a trained nurse and Hospital things, but I want you to look him up.

There is much more to William Worth's story. At 5 foot 10 inches tall, with a fair complexion, hazel eyes, and brown hair, the 20-year-old trainee engine driver enlisted early, within one month of war being declared. Like

Wilfred Hartridge, William was a private in the 3rd Battalion and took part in the Gallipoli landing on 25 April 1915. He lasted three weeks. On 19 May, during a major Turkish attack, William was shot through the neck. The bullet entered the left side of his neck, passing through his back, and exiting through the eighth scapula. He was completely paralysed. It took five days for Worth to be evacuated, arriving in Malta on 25 May. He was admitted to Valletta Hospital with the most serious cases, into Ward C where Narrelle had just started working. Worth was therefore one of Narrelle's first patients and his condition profoundly affected her. The young, vulnerable and desperately ill soldier became a favourite, not only because of his dire medical condition but also because of his endearing, gentle, and uncomplaining personality.

Worth sent a cable to his recently widowed mother saying he was 'slightly wounded doing well', which was a complete understatement. He then asked Narrelle if she could write a letter to her. Narrelle was most happy to oblige the young patient and on 31 May, an emotional Narrelle wrote to Edith Worth.

Dear Mrs Worth,

Your son asked if I would write and tell you he is in this Hospital.

He has been rather badly wounded in his shoulder, the right shoulder blade being severely shattered, he also has partial paralysis of the whole body & is slightly deaf, but we have every hope for his recovery, especially as he is giving himself every chance, by not worrying.

He is quite my best patient, never grumbles or complains and is so grateful for anything we do for him, and my one regret is, that I have not time, with all my other patients, to do everything I would like to do, for them all, When you write to him do not mention his paralysis, he asked me not to tell you, his words were 'Tell Mother about me Sister but make it as OK & bright & hopeful as you can, don't tell her about my old limbs', which made me nearly cry, but that is just what he is like in the ward, he will often say 'Do the next boy first Sister he is worse than I am'.

Oh, you Mothers you must be proud of your sons, they are splendid, the things they have done & the way they stand their pain. I am an Australian myself, & only came over last month from New South Wales.

I shall hope to be able to report good progress from time to time, & when you write your son just be as cheery as you can, but of course, I was forgetting how long it will be before you get this. I hope that by that time he will be well enough to be moved to a convalescence Hospital, he is so glad to think he has done his 'little bit' and wants to 'get better to have another shot at them', meaning the Turks.

Your son sends all kinds of good wishes to you and hopes you are quite well. With kindest regards, trusting I will be able to give you better news some other time.

Yours truly, Sister N. Hobbes.

Narrelle continued to correspond with William's mother. On 21 July she sent another letter to Edith, updating her on her son's condition, particularly concerned that William has received no letters from his mother, or indeed anyone, since his arrival.

I've really intended writing you quite often about your son, but have been so busy, and have had such numbers of letters to write that I am afraid I did not realise how time was flying, and that you would be anxiously waiting for news of the wounded one.

He is getting on splendidly, and can now lift his feet up & find his way to his mouth, with a little trouble, but we feel certain that with time and massage he will quite regain the use of his limbs, and he has never given up hope, sometimes he gets a little bit doubtful about things I think for he gets so quiet, but mostly he is very cheerful.

He is a great favourite with all in the Hospital, and we shall all miss him very much when we send him back to you in Australia, we do not know when that will be, but as soon as there is a hospital boat running out there, you see he will be unfit for further active service, any way for a very long time, and they are not sending any, unfit for further service, to England. He is very anxious to know how you are, and is always wondering when he will hear from you, he has had no letters at all since he has been in here, or for some time before.

Worthie sends his love to you all, and to all the children.

We have such numbers of Australian soldiers in this Hospital and I think they like having an Australian Sister in the ward.

With very kindest regards.

Yours sincerely (Sister) Narrelle Hobbes

After being stabilised in Malta, William Worth, or 'Worthie' as he was known on the ward, was evacuated to England on 6 August on the

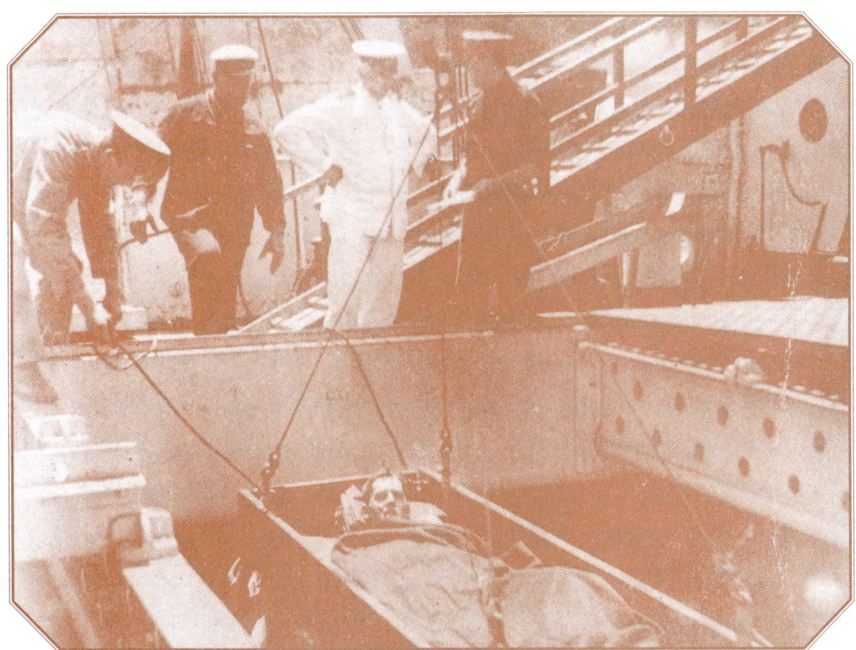

Private William Worth, totally paralysed from a bullet wound, was one of Narrelle's favourite patients. Here he is embarking on the *Glengorm Castle*, 6 August 1915. *(Worth Papers, Mitchell Library, Sydney)*

Glengorm Castle. He was admitted to Wandsworth Hospital in London, and later spent time in specialist rehabilitation in Essex. Despite Narrelle thinking he would immediately be sent back to Australia, it took almost a year for him to return home.

In November, while still in Malta, Narrelle received a letter from Worth. She was so excited because he had written it himself, and *he always said that if ever he was able to write, his first letter would be to me*. Narrelle immediately wrote back to him.

> *Worthie dear I was most awfully pleased to get your letter the other day, I simply cannot tell you how rejoiced I am to hear that you have got on as well, why I was able to read your letter quite well, with the exception of the address, I'm not quite sure of that, and won't your Mother be pleased, I had a most charming letter from her some time ago and if I can find it I will send it on to you.*
>
> *Of course you could not help but get better over there in beautiful England but all the same won't it be glorious to find yourself steaming up Sydney harbour … do you remember little Ken Williams, the boy who was paralysed from his hips? I had a letter the other day from a chum of his, saying they had operated on him the day before and had extracted the bullet from the spine, and had every hope that he would be able to walk about again. Isn't it splendid, I got his letter the same day I got yours, and was tremendously excited over them both, as you can imagine.*
>
> *… Goodnight, write me again someday. I need not tell you how delighted I shall be to hear from you at any time … With very kindest regards and all good wishes for a happy Xmas and a speedy & safe return to dear old Australia.*
>
> *Yours very sincerely,*
>
> *Narrelle Hobbes*

This important milestone was matched by the news that William could now walk, with the aid of a stick, which made Narrelle very happy, although she confided to her family, *of course I am simply delighted tho it will be months and months before he can do anything ever*. William was invalided back to Australia on 8 May 1916, and discharged from the army. He spent time in Randwick Hospital undergoing further rehabilitation. In 1917, he was living in Granville receiving a pension of £3 a fortnight, permanently scarred from his war experience and uncertain if he could ever hold down a job. He was only 23 years old.

However, despite all the odds, William Worth's story has a happy ending. His physical recovery was such that although his legs and hands were permanently affected, he was able to find employment as a clerk at Victoria Barracks in Sydney. There, in 1921, he met Joan Butler, who worked as a stenographer and typist in the Intelligence Section and was a cousin of Charles Bean, the war correspondent, and his brothers Jack and Monty. After a three-year courtship, William and Joan married, moved to Roseville on Sydney's North Shore, and had one daughter. Despite being a TPI (Totally and Permanently Incapacitated), William Worth managed to overcome his war disabilities to lead a productive life, involving himself in organisations such as the Gallipoli Legion Bowling Club and the Millions Club. He died in the early 1980s.

War was a lottery and Narrelle was beginning to realise that fact. There was no way of knowing what was going to happen, or what the fate of her patients would be. She developed a close bond with many of them, a bond that would last her lifetime. Not only did Narrelle feel the full force of the wartime experiences of her patients, but her family and friends became directly involved too. Narrelle had male cousins who had enlisted in the AIF, including Gilbert Goldie Anschau. Growing up in different parts of New South Wales, Narrelle and Gilbert had not seen much of each other. It was through war that their paths crossed again. Narrelle met up with Gilbert at the Imtarfa Hospital, Malta.

He arrived there on 31 August from Gallipoli with enteric fever. Imtarfa Hospital was perched high up in the middle of the island away from everyone, but able to catch the breeze. Originally it was to be used for venereal disease patients from Egypt but once the Gallipoli campaign was underway, it became the main hospital for dysentery and other infectious diseases. It was always full to capacity.

Gilbert, from Lismore in northern New South Wales, was 27 years old, single, and a clerk in Public Works when he enlisted as a stretcher bearer in the 1st Field Ambulance. Like many of Narrelle's patients, he was part of the original landing on Gallipoli on 25 April. He was a handsome and popular man; of average height, 5 foot 9¾ inches tall, thick set, with dark hair, brown eyes, a fair complexion and moustache. Once Gilbert was better, Narrelle had hoped to do some sightseeing to Citta Vecchia with him but as she explained to her family,

> *We were going to explore things together if I could get a holiday & he could get out of hospital instead of which he rang up on Wed to say goodbye, he was being sent on to England. I was so disappointed … poor boy he was simply delighted to see me the afternoon I went out to him was quite excited — I went out the day I sent the p.c.* [postcard] *a few days before but he had just gone away from the ward & they couldn't find him & as it was getting late & the last train!!! left at 7.30pm. I couldn't wait & I had a most pathetic letter from him a few days later saying how sorry he was he had missed me & as I had said I'd go out again in a few days he wouldn't budge away from the ward again till he saw me. So when I got a holiday I went out, such a long way to go from here & the trains only run every hour but a beautiful position — he didn't have Enteric but dysentery now he has gone to England — am afraid they'd have a rotten trip too there is a perfect gale blowing, poor dears.*

Gilbert Anschau was admitted to Netley Hospital in October 1915 and later returned to Australia. After spending time with his family — his mother, Ruth and father John, who was the postmaster at Parramatta, and his younger brother and sister — Gilbert re-enlisted in the 3rd Battalion of the AIF as a corporal. Once more he sailed out of Sydney, on 7 October 1916, this time on the HMAT *Ceramic* as part of the 21st reinforcements. Arriving in France in February 1917, Gilbert Anschau was involved in the two battles for Bullecourt in April and May 1917. Slightly wounded on 17 April, he returned to his unit, only to be killed on 5 May 1917, two days into the second battle of Bullecourt. These battles were so intense and the fighting conditions so appalling that we can only imagine what the soldiers on all sides — Australians, British and Germans — endured.

Bullecourt is viewed by historians as a costly and largely unnecessary battle in which thousands of Australian soldiers were butchered through inept British strategy under General Hubert Gough. Even Charles Bean conceded that Bullecourt 'more than any other battle, shook the confidence of Australian soldiers in the capacity of the British command'. Part of flanking operations around the small French town of Bullecourt, the Australians were generally fighting in open countryside that had become a muddy quagmire due to the constant and relentless bombardment by the artillery.

Gilbert Anschau was not reported wounded and missing until 11 May, one week after his death, and was only confirmed killed in action in September, four months later. His official file states that Gilbert was buried in the vicinity of Maricourt Wood, but that is not quite true. Along with 2423 other Australian soldiers who went missing on the Bullecourt battlefield, Gilbert's body was never found. It simply disappeared into the muddy wasteland that was the western front in 1917.

No-one, especially the Australian authorities, really knew what had happened to him. Gilbert's family was, understandably, desperately worried. The only information they received from the army was a couple of brief telegrams. The original one simply stated that their son was reported missing and wounded, somewhere in France. *Should any further particulars be received you will be informed immediately* it concluded in the military's perfunctory style. It was not until months later that Gilbert was confirmed dead but no identity discs were supplied to the grieving family. This was, of course, because there was no body, but the authorities could not tell the family that. Gilbert's father wrote repeatedly to the army asking for some sort of tangible, physical verification of his son's death. But to no avail.

The Anschaus then turned to the Australian Red Cross Society. Their Wounded and Missing Enquiry Bureau was often the last resort for distraught families. The Bureau had branches in each Australian state as well as a London office, run by 24-year-old Vera Deakin, daughter of Alfred Deakin. It supplied information on missing, sick and wounded Australian soldiers in all theatres of the war. The Red Cross had searchers in the field and good contacts with the Australian military, as well as teams of investigators back home. A Red Cross report in October 1917 stated that Gilbert Anschau was a machine gunner and had been wounded in the eye. He headed off to a dressing station which was over open country and extremely dangerous to traverse. He was not seen again. Later an eyewitness account added more information to Gilbert's last moments.

> *I was in the same trench with him in front of Bullecourt and he was standing on the fire step and was shot through the eye by a sniper. He made an exclamation and immediately went over the top and had gone about 500 yards towards the German line when he was blown to pieces by a shell.*

This eyewitness, Private Philip Ottaway, a 24-year-old blacksmith from rural New South Wales, gave his testimony from his hospital bed in Birmingham, England. He was suffering from a severe case of endemic trench fever (contracted from lice). Ottaway was later discharged with nephritis, a renal disease common in the trenches, and invalided back to Australia.

Gilbert's sister, Miss B. Anschau, from the Domestic Science School at Parramatta, wrote to the authorities in the early 1920s asking where her brother was buried as she was planning a trip to France and wanted to visit his grave. Of course, there was no grave and no identifiable graveyard for her to visit. Miss Anschau would have to wait until 1938 when the

Villers–Bretonneaux Memorial was opened. There she would have seen her brother's name etched into the white stone walls — Corporal Gilbert Goldie Anschau, 3rd Battalion — along with the names of the 10,700 other Australian soldiers who died in the Somme and Arras area who have no known grave. In simple terms they all, like Gilbert Anschau, were blown to pieces or buried under tonnes of rich, fertile French soil, never to be found.

BUT THIS WAS ALL IN THE FUTURE. AUSTRALIAN TROOPS WERE NOT EVEN in France in September 1915. Narrelle was not to know that on that hot, hot day in Malta when she had the day off and travelled out to the Imfarta Hospital to catch up with her cousin that he would have already been moved off the island, and that she would never see him again.

War was like that. One minute you would meet up with someone, the next they would be a name on a casualty list or worse. Narrelle was learning fast how transitory military life could be. It was all part of being on active service.

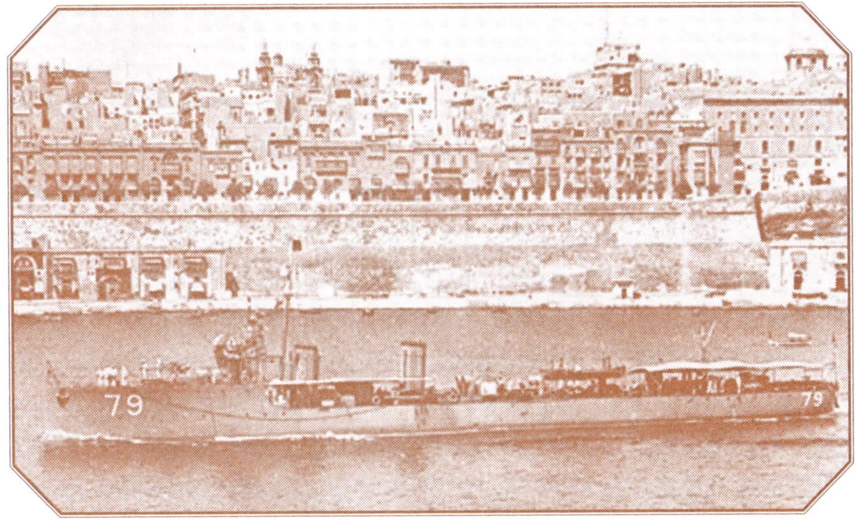

Valletta Harbour (H12463: *Australian War Memorial*)

Chapter 4

'DEAR, DIRTY, NOISY, ADORABLE MALTA'

JUST AS NARRELLE WAS ADJUSTING TO BEING ON ACTIVE SERVICE, SHE, too, was getting used to Malta. She had never experienced a place quite like it and it was a culture shock for the girl from the Australian bush. Narrelle often described her reactions to Malta and the Maltese in her letters home, especially the different customs such as the Southern European practice of closing the shops from 1 till 3 for 'siesta'. This was a very sensible idea, Narrelle thought, when the sirocco was blowing and the intense summer heat was overbearing. She liked nothing better than to come off duty, tear off her layers of clothing — apron, dress and petticoat — take down her hair, lie in her underclothes under a fan, and sleep.

Narrelle was also amused by the abundance of goats that wandered through the dusty, narrow streets of Valletta with the goat tenderer yelling 'milk' at the top of his voice. As a country girl, she was used to milking dairy cows and knew how it was done, but this was a new experience for her. She explained how once a customer was found, the goat herder would stop the herd in the street and milk the goats, sometimes ten or twelve of them, straight into the customer's jugs and pots, and then haggle for a price, another foreign custom.

The nurses were instructed not to drink the goat's milk because of the fear that it spread fever, so tinned milk from England was made available to all medical staff. Indeed, according to Narrelle, the food generally on Malta was not terribly good. Sometimes the nurses took themselves off for a treat in the one local restaurant considered suitable for them. As Narrelle explained:

> *Talking about being different, this is the very funniest place I've ever been into. You wander down the middle of the narrow streets and — oh let me tell you what we have for afternoon tea when we go out for it, which we often do if two or three of us are off together, we go out and feed, we do not get good meals here, sometimes they are very off in fact, so we go and have bacon and eggs, toast or rolls and ice cream, at the only place in town we are allowed to dine. There is only one eating place in Valletta where we are allowed to eat, for fear of Mediterranean fever, typhoid or cholera, so needless to say we are careful.*

The heat of the summer months and the close living, antiquated sewerage and low levels of hygiene all made an impression on Narrelle, not always positive. In a letter to sister Kit, Narrelle again tried to explain her reaction to, and impressions of, Valletta.

> *It's not a bad sort of place, after 6.30pm then the quaintness & strangeness & even the beauty of it shows up, but it is all so fearfully built in, with its walls & rocks. You look over a wall & see the spot you want to get to just a few feet below, but to get there you have to go round & round & up & down, because you are simply 'shut in'. I'd try & describe some of the places I like most, old forts etc, but if the censor read it he would probably gum it all down or return it, or burn it, and we can't send post cards of the most interesting places, so they also are forbidden such a pity.*

Steeped in history, Narrelle found her surroundings fascinating. Although the myriad church bells were silenced by British military authorities on appeal to the Archbishop of Malta, everywhere she turned there was a fascinating array of historical sites in the bustling and congested town. In a letter written in early July to her niece Joan Commons, Narrelle provided a potted history lesson.

> *Malta is a most weird place, very interesting, it's so* <u>*very*</u> *ancient. Saint Paul is supposed to have been ship wrecked here, & some of the buildings, a great many of them in fact, date back to 1500 & something. This Hospital* [Valletta Hospital] *dates back to the Knights of St John. I can't describe the houses to you, for the simple reason they are all square & all run one into the other, all have flat roofs, & high stone walls to keep you from falling out. You look over one side & look down about 100 feet or more, 200, go to the other side & look over & you find yourself on the next man's roof. All the clothes are dried up there or out of the windows on lines, I often wonder if* [how] *ours are dried & washed. All the walls are about 3 ft deep, when you go out, you mostly walk down the middle of the street, only getting out of the way of Caroggies cab (pronounced carotze) and garlicky Maltese.*

When she had time off, Narrelle also enjoyed browsing and shopping. She especially liked the Maltese lace, made famous in the mid-nineteenth century with its geometric patterns of Maltese crosses and small ears of wheat. As Maltese lace was well known, her mother and sisters inquired about it. Narrelle responded:

> *Yes you can get Maltese lace linen & insertions for anything from 3/6 a piece of 6–7 yards they sell it in bundles of 6–7 yards. I got a perfectly sweet piece the other day about 3 inches wide 6 & three quarter yards for 6/-. You can get it any width insertion with lace to match some of it at 2/- & 2/6 a yard is exquisite about 4 inches wide & table centres quite large for 18/- simply beautiful.*

It was this kind of simple exchanging of information between mother and daughter, and between sisters and friends, about mundane, everyday topics that sustained Narrelle during her war service. The importance of communication home cannot be underestimated. Both the receiving and writing of letters dominated her life. Despite her best efforts, Narrelle was often lonely and desperately homesick. Letters therefore became her lifeline to a once familiar world outside the military and medical madness that was Malta in the summer of 1915. Narrelle often talked in her letters about the importance of receiving mail, which was infrequent and haphazard. It affected her moods and could make her quite depressed or elated depending on the circumstances. On 12 July, she confided to her family:

Oh darlings I sort of don't know where to begin, such a mail day, I've not had any letters for nearly a fortnight. Of course we are very lucky to get letters the way we do considering we are on active service and it's war time, but one does so long for something that is right from home, even if there is absolutely no news in it. Well to-day over in the ward I said to the Sister working with me, 'I should give just anything I could to go over to the Camaretta to dinner and find an Australian mail for me there', and lo, as I crossed the street I saw three sisters standing up the stairs shaking their fists at me and saying 'you mean thing the whole mail is for you'. I made one bound and tore round the balcony as tho I had been shot from a gun, and there was a pile of letters. I could not believe they were really all for me, till the Home Sister said 'You need not go through them Sister they are all yours'. I bounded into the dining room to see how many Els and Rose had and ran into Matron who said it looked as tho I needed a day off duty and an orderly to carry up my mail. I could hardly bother having any dinner, but guessed that by the time I had finished reading I would be ready for food, so sat and ate food, and then came to my room, undressed, and got just into bloomers and singlet (of the thinnest), before I opened one letter, took my hair down so the perspiration could dry, threw myself on the bed and devoured letters, 14, oh scrummie … I did rejoice, ever so many thanks dears, you simply don't know how letters are appreciated just now, and we hear simply no Australian news.

Not only was Narrelle starved of news from home and homesick but so, too, were her patients. William Worth, for example, the soldier paralysed from the neck down, received no letters from home whilst in her care, and this deeply concerned Narrelle. She was always asking her family to send over old newspapers, journals, anything that the 'boys' could read to remind them of home. Narrelle noted that her patients did not want news of the war. Rather they were desperate for news of Australia and home that specifically did *not* mention the war.

> *Many thanks for papers the boys love them several have said quite pathetically to me 'Sister I wish they would print a paper for us chaps at the front without any war news, unless it's the casualty list — give us some Australian New South Wales scenes to look at instead of war pictures like our own country would be alright — we've seen shells burst & dead turks & comrades enough to last for the rest of our lives in reality'.*

Narrelle also encouraged her family to motivate people back in Australia to write to 'A wounded Australian soldier' just so that they would feel cared for and wanted. In a letter to Els written on 17 July, Narrelle concluded:

> *Ocean of love dearies all, and write often, and tell me all you hear, we get <u>no</u> news more often than not and what we hear is not always reliable and <u>do</u> send some Australian papers, get some of your friends to, and tell them also, the men love getting letters, they have been getting some addressed to 'A wounded Australian soldier' Military Hospital, Malta — or Egypt as the case may be. They love them, filled with all sorts of Australian news, from men, women and children, and on the top of the envelope is written 'Please give this to someone who does not get any letters'. I've several in my ward and they are passed on from ward to ward, till sometimes they come to a man who has been wanting news of people and places.*

Not surprisingly, Narrelle developed close relationships with her patients. She became particularly involved with certain ones such as William Worth, who was a special favourite. Being subjected to war not only brought soldiers together through shared experiences, but also the nurses. They were all on active service together, both nurse and soldier. Many wrote letters to Narrelle after they had either been sent back to Gallipoli or evacuated to England.

> *I've had such a crowd of letters lately from patients who have gone to England — I love to hear how they are when they leave here & some of them are such dears — but I must confess there are times when I have to puzzle out just who they are — it's almost impossible to keep track of names & patients.*

It was particularly hard when soldiers recovered from their wounds or illness and returned to Gallipoli. Narrelle hated the idea of nursing the men back to health in order for them to embark again for the peninsula. *We've just been sending such a crowd of boys back to the front it makes one very sad to see them going back to it all — not so bad when they go over 1st but to have to go back to it.* This was a particular dilemma faced by all medical staff in war: to patch someone up in order for him to return to the front line to be possibly hurt again or disfigured, or even killed.

Narrelle was also particularly keen to nurse Australian and New Zealand men, and referred to them as 'my boys'. This was what she had enlisted for in the first place and her active service in Malta, despite all the problems and hard work, provided her with that opportunity. She did not care where she was sent, as long as she nursed Australian patients. Not only did she nurse them but she clearly spent considerable time, effort and money providing them with little extras to make their life better. She also shared that sense of humour peculiar to the Australians, and enjoyed joking with them.

> *We've really had some awfully nice boys in just lately — I've pledged*

myself to buy all sorts of things when he [a soldier] *sends over some money — & gives me the address of his various people. Another boy has promised a badge of every Regt. in N.Z. which I shall simply adore — for some of them are beautiful — one nice Australian presented me with his only badge to wear, so that the Australians would recognise me at once as one — they were having a heated argument in one tent yesterday as to whether I was English or Australian. Then when I got to the next tent there was a Queenslander with a most beautiful Emu plume in his hat so I said to the Sister 'Look Sister are not these Kangaroo feathers beautiful — they are kangaroo feathers are they not?' He looked at me for a moment as much as to say ye gods you blithering idiot & then I could see he felt sorry for my ignorance for he said quite quietly 'No Sister not kangaroo but "Emu"'. Oh Emu I said what's an Emu like? I always thought they were kangaroo feathers — he sighed & said quite patiently 'No Sister, a Kangaroo is an animal with fur but an Emu is a bird like an Ostrich'. After I passed I heard him say to an Australian near him isn't it wonderful how little these English people* [know] *about Australia & the Australians. So this afternoon I'm going to arm myself with some Australian papers & take them to the tent & tell him I'm an Australian.*

Her 'boys' clearly became very fond of Narrelle too. Their friendships, whilst largely transient, were important for both nurse and patient. For example Narrelle told the story of the night she went to the Italian Opera, *La Bohème*, and then had to attend an 'At Home' at Government House: *... we do so hate them, absolutely the very stodgiest 'do' you could imagine.* Narrelle fell ill with a bad head cold, and had the next day off duty. As she continued:

... that night just before supper one of the Sisters came up to my room with a note in one hand and a most beautiful bunch of roses in the other. One of my naughty Australian boys had heard I was sick and nicked out and bought them for me, wasn't it sweet of him. They are such dears,

> *they are very naughty tho but I love them all. Today I was in a tent talking to some, both English and Australian. One little A*[ustralian] *boy, full of mischief most times was a bit depressed and I just stopped to speak to him, and something came up about a boy who had died, and this youngster said 'Oh well you know Sister you can only die once, and one might as well die here as in Gallipoli, I wouldn't be missed much wherever I died' and when I turned round to speak to him his eyes were full up and he could not answer me, but pretended to be laughing. I just felt I wanted to sit down and talk to him there and then, instead of which someone came for me and I had to leave him to it.*

ANOTHER MAIN THEME OF NARRELLE'S WARTIME CORRESPONDENCE WAS the general treatment of nurses by the military. She found the restrictions and rules of the British military nursing service very hard to understand, and difficult to adhere to, and she railed against them regularly in her letters home. Whilst she appreciated and understood the discipline necessary for general nursing, Narrelle was particularly annoyed by the lack of personal freedom in the military.

> *We are not allowed to wear any blessed article of clothing that is not uniform, and we* <u>*are*</u> *getting so sick of it, and yearn to get into a cool white dress, & a shady hat with one or two jolly flowers on it. We three* [Narrelle, Elsie Welman and Rose Kirkaldie] *sold nearly all our clothing before we left London. It was no use putting it away for months & months, for goodness knows* <u>*when*</u> *we will wear private clothing again, & by the time we get back to London our things will be moth-eaten & old fashioned, so we just sold them.*

Narrelle found it challenging to say the least, to be a civilian one day, and then thrust into the military the next. She was an independent woman who was used to controlling her own life. The conventions of military life and the status of different groups within the army irritated her with an intensity that grew during her war service. Being an Australian — and a colonial — within the British nursing service, provided Narrelle with particular difficulties that she had not thought about before joining up. It was the strict fraternisation rules imposed on nurses between male nursing staff (or any men, officers and soldiers included for that matter), and the differentiation between officers and soldiers that especially irked Narrelle. These rules and regulations were generally enforced more rigorously in the British services. As she exploded to her family:

> *It was quite a knotty problem among the matrons because one of the VAD girls discovered her brother on the island, he was a private in the AIF & she had to get special leave to see him. Guess I'd say be D_____ to such rules if I met my brother or any one else I was keen about. They should remember this is a very different army to Regular army, it's purely volunteers and there are as good and better men in the ranks as among the officers.*

She also blamed many of the problems on the behaviour of certain nurses:

> *We are not allowed to have anything to do with the orderlies beyond the ward work, & must not stand & speak to one outside our wards … the rule is being enforced because I believe some of the Sisters are by way of making fools of themselves with some of the orderlies, mind you … some of them* [orderlies] *are awful fools. Look I'd rather be born a woman 5 times over than be a man like some of the men I've come across out here, blithering idiots with as many brains as a cabbage. Tell an ordinary pro the same thing for two mornings running & she remembers it, tell the average Tommy orderly the same thing two mornings running — & you keep right on telling him.*

This unflattering view of the RAMC orderlies was carried over into Narrelle's comparisons between English and Australian soldiers. She was always comparing them. For example in a letter dated 10 July, she wrote to her family extolling and romanticising the virtues of Australians and Australian soldiers.

> *Oh they are great little people are the people of our island, and yet the Australian men get blamed for everything that is done, simply because they do things openly and don't mind if they are found out, while the English Tommies do things behind the Officers backs and don't get found out, and then the Australians are blamed for it. But all the same I'm jolly proud of being an Australian, they are splendid.*

During the war this was a common theme with Australian soldiers and much has been written about the Anzacs as a volunteer force: their lampooning of British officers, their unwillingness to kowtow to authority, and their innate belief that Australians (or colonials) were better than the Tommy soldiers. Attitudes of egalitarianism and non-acceptance of class are also part of this peculiarly Australian behaviour, which is generally attributed to Australian men *not* Australian women, and especially not nurses. Yet in Narrelle's case, this 'larrikin streak' or lack of deference to authority figures was clearly evident throughout her correspondence. Her sense of being different from the British because she was an Australian developed early on in her military career, and from the outset, on board the *Mongolia* as she sailed towards Malta, Narrelle believed that Australian nurses were better trained and generally superior to their British equivalents.

Narrelle also used her letters home as a way of venting her anger and frustration at the challenging and, in her eyes, questionable nursing practices she was exposed to on Malta. She wrote a long, detailed, seething letter on 23 July to her close nursing friend and mate, Smithie. After two months of active service, with little respite, where she was constantly challenged by the job, Narrelle was feeling the strain. Her intolerant streak was in evidence. She tried to explain it all to her friend.

My dearest Smithkins,

I don't owe you a letter but I want to get some things off my chest and as you are a nurse, you would understand things a bit better than a non nurse, but even you dear could not understand half the things I want to talk over, no-one could who had not been in a Military Hospital in war time. Stay where you are my dear, stay right there, &, if you must, look after the men we are sending, &, for god's sake make up to them for all they have gone through over this side. I'm in a bad temper today, and could howl over the patheticness [sic] *of some of the cases up in this division, and when I think of all they have gone through, and all they have given up for this, good lord.*

... I wish I could just chuck everything off my chest, including the Maltese Drs, that our men are obliged to be looked after by, some of them is damnable, absolutely, when there are so many good men knocking around, they don't know anything and won't admit that they don't. They are like a lot of jabbering monkeys, of course the poor souls it's not altogether their fault, they can't get the experience here. Thank goodness I've got the best M.O. [medical officer] *in the Hospital in my wards, but Smithie it's very heartbreaking work at times, and sometimes we three can't help thinking that the life of a man is of no account really, as long as you do not have a mistake in your diet sheet, or the amount of kit in the wards, &, if you want to learn new* methods *of treatment* STAY WHERE YOU ARE IN THE BACKBLOCKS.

... I must stop now, we are getting new patients in today, pretty sick ones I believe, especially Enteric, it's broken out over there, isn't it awful ... Good night dear, don't mind this outburst, I think I'll try & get on a Hospital ship, some of our Sisters have gone on them already.

Oceans of love from your old mate.

NARRELLE WAS NOT TRANSFERRED TO A HOSPITAL SHIP. RATHER, SHE WAS promoted. She was, after all, a capable nurse, intelligent, adaptable, organised, and quick to learn. Despite her forthright opinions, which she, perhaps wisely, largely kept to herself, her talents were clearly visible to her superiors. In August 1915, Narrelle was asked by her matron if she would take charge of St David's Camp. St David's was a new hospital with 1000 beds constructed on the ridge above Valletta. It was built entirely of white canvas tents. Located to catch the breeze, it was considerably cooler than the stifling conditions in Valletta during summer. The request had come from Jane Hoadley, the matron in charge of all nursing staff on Malta, so Narrelle could hardly refuse. However, she was not very pleased about it, as she related to her family.

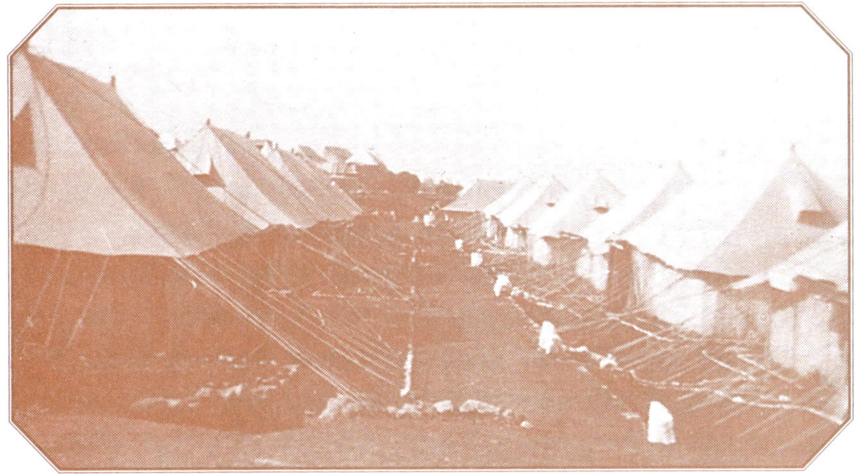

St David's Tent Hospital, Malta, 1915. (*Hobbes Collection*)

25th August 1915.
My very dearest Peoples,

Yes here I am, doing Camp life and when I try in my mind's eye to think how to describe it to you words fail me. You simply cannot imagine what its like. I don't know just where to begin there is so much to write about & tell you that everything gets into a sort of jumbled mass, & my brain

& feet ache too much to sort things out. Last Sunday week Matron came to me about 7.30pm & said 'Sister I have to send you out to St David's Camp to take charge till you can get things running properly. Miss Hoadley came to me & asked if I had a Sister I could send out in charge, one I could recommend, who had some method, the Sisters she sent out seemed to have no method, and no idea how to manage, the place was in an absolute muddle & the C.O. nearly frantic & I told Miss Hoadley I thought you could do it, easily. You will go over in an ambulance in the morning & come back each night till we can make the arrangements'. Of course I nearly wept on the spot as I had just got my wards into good running order & four days before, I had got a new batch of men, awfully bad cases, & I was having the time of my life, going like mad, and then to have to give it up & go to the camp, simply because the idiots of English sisters had not enough brain power to work out a thing and make the work run smoothly. Really they drive me to distraction most of them, I've never met such a brainless crowd of women as we have out here.

Well I came out, I saw, and then sat down in my tent to try & grasp things. There are 78 large tents for Hospital, containing 1000 beds; and swarms of other tents, the 78 all hold from 12 to 16 patients, there are about 12 medical men and 6 sisters (self included), so you can imagine how we go … I've never been so desperately homesick in all my life. I hate being here but I like being at the Camp in the day. The sad part of it is Matron came to me the other day and asked when I thought I would be able to come back, she was in despair about my ward, it was in a most frantic muddle. I was furious, but it was only another result of the dear English sisters methods, and I don't care now if I don't go back to it, I seem to spend my time lately straightening things out for the idiots to muddle up. I get so mad, and I suppose just when I get things going out here I'll be yanked off to some other blooming place, however it's all in a lifetime. There are hundreds of dear Australian lads out there at the Camp, and we are sending such crowds of them to England, they love getting there and get so excited when the list goes round of the men who are to go that day …

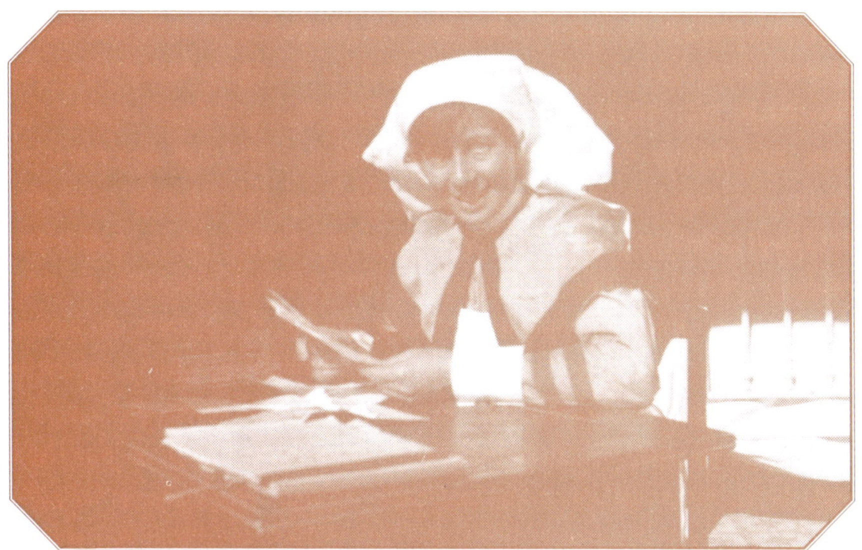

Narrelle as Matron of St David's, Malta, 1915. (*Haskins Collection*)

> *Dear 'little' Tonie* [Hordern] *went back to the Dardanelles last week. He came to say good-bye to me, you might ring his mother up will you, I would write to her but have not time really. He looked well but very thin, and I would have liked to have seen him looking a bit better. He was very glad to get back, did not like Pembroke and I do not wonder at it, it's just across the road from us … I had a p.c. from Holt* [Hardy] *and a letter from Wilfred Hartridge who said if he is ever brought to Malta he will demand to be brought to my ward and refuse to go anywhere else …* [Narrelle was not to know that Wilfred was already dead, killed two weeks earlier on Gallipoli.]

Considerable voluntary help was provided to the twenty hospitals and their thousands of patients and staff by the British Red Cross through their Joint War Committee and the ladies committee established on Malta by Lady Methuen. As the size and scale of the medical facilities on Malta increased, with the opening of additional hospitals such as St David's, the patriotic funds had to work that much harder. Three Red Cross commissioners — the aptly named Captain Stockings, Mr Tindal Robertson and Lieutenant Colonel Ashley — were despatched to the island to assist with co-ordination and administration of supplies. As the patients were coming directly from the Gallipoli peninsula, they did not bring much with them. Volunteer workers met each ship and provided drinks to the patients as they waited to be offloaded, assessed, and directed to the various hospitals. Each patient who arrived on the island was provided with a parcel of stationery, tobacco and matches, as well as pyjamas, shirts and socks.

One of the main wartime tasks for women left at home in Australia was to become involved in patriotic funds. There were literally hundreds of different funds of various size and focus established during the war. For example, the Sandbag List Fund raised money for sandbags to be sent to Gallipoli; the Blue Cross Fund assisted the horses left behind in Egypt; and the Army Bands Fund purchased musical instruments. But the largest patriotic funds of the war included the Salvation Army, the Australian Comforts Fund and the Australian Red Cross, and it was these organisations that raised most of the £14 million which was eventually donated by the Australian population. Before the creation of the Department of Repatriation in late 1917, state-based patriotic funds, such as the Lord Mayor's Patriotic Fund in New South Wales, largely managed the stipends and allowances for soldiers' dependents and returned soldiers.

The knitting of socks epitomised women's voluntary wartime work. From the coalface, Narrelle encouraged this endeavour. In a letter dated 5 October, she wrote, *Sox my dear — you keep right on knitting them — you should see some of the fellows these boys are issued with, they boil them at the laundry or do some other fool thing — anyway they come back with the foot about 4 inches long simply awful. You can't send too many socks for them.*

There was a certain amount of self-regulation amongst the patriotic funds. The Red Cross provided assistance to the sick and wounded soldiers, whilst the Salvation Army, Australian Comforts Fund and

YMCA looked after the fit and well soldiers. In Malta, there was quite a deal of overlapping. For example, the Australian Red Cross donated £2000 to build a large stone auditorium between St Andrew's and St Paul's hospitals that could seat 2000 for concerts. The building was opened by Lord Methuen in January 1916. It still exists today and is in the process of being renovated. The Salvation Army and YMCA, as well as other local Maltese voluntary organisations, established tea rooms, and organised sporting games and other recreational pursuits in order to prevent men from visiting the bordellos and drinking houses which, typical of all seafaring ports, flourished in Malta. Narrelle mentioned this problem indirectly in one of her letters but, as always, she sided with the Australians.

> *I had another of the Yeomans in, a cousin* [Sydney Ernest Yeomans] *(45-ish I imagine). He is now doing 21 days for going out of Hospital & getting drunk, and that's another thing on my chest, the thousands of men on this island, who get a pass from the Dr & go out, and, well it's not right to let them just wander around, getting into all manner of mischief, either drinking, tho they are not supposed to touch it, and are only given 2/- a week, but you can get a bottle of Malta wine for 7d or less, but I'm afraid they are going to have trouble here if the men are not kept down a bit, and the New Z's & Australians are getting the blame for a good deal. Mind you, they are not by any means always the ringleaders.*

BY OCTOBER 1915, NARRELLE WAS STILL MATRON OF ST DAVID'S. SHE was beginning to flag under the continuous, unabated, arduous workload. The hospital was vast and spread out. She and the other nursing staff spent their shifts moving from tent to tent, tending to their patients. Narrelle found it quite exhausting. Because the hospital was virtually in the open air, she found herself going very brown, or tanned, when such a condition was not considered either ladylike or

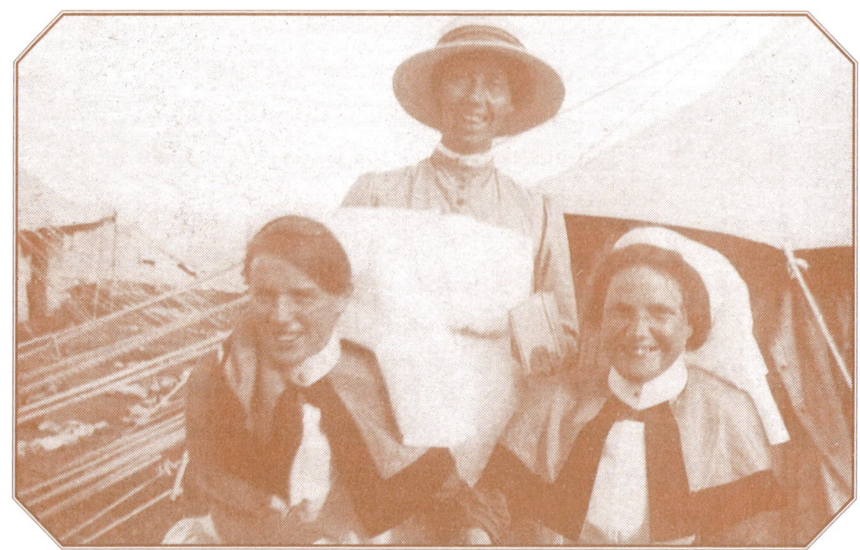

Narrelle and two sisters, St David's, Malta, 1915. (*Hobbes Collection*)

appropriate. *We camp sisters are going absolutely black, I'm nearly the colour of my suitcase. When we get back to London we will have to enter a convent or something for a few months & undergo a face peeling treatment*, she explained in a letter home. Narrelle had been on Malta for five months, with only the odd day off in all that time. There was no respite for her and the other nurses and medical staff from the gruelling job of wartime nursing. The physical conditions of her work environment were poor, and whilst the heat of the Maltese summer had abated the sirocco had not, as she unburdened herself, once more, to her family in a letter dated 13 October 1915.

> *Darlings, I meant to write quite a long letter today, but the flesh is weak & the Sirrocco is bad! My blood has turned to water, & my bones to powder, I am a jelly or any other old thing — Honestly this Sirrocco business is most 'impolite' eh what! When I wakened this morning my clothes and everything in the room was wet like a mist rain that did not fall over the island but is not hot. That is in the ordinary way. It is like going into one of the hot houses in the gardens. At night as soon as the sun*

goes down, it gets quite cold and we have to put on our coats, everything is damp, the sugar is like damp salt and sweets get wet and sticky. Oh, this is some place I assure you. What! I wish this damnable war would end, but there seems as much chance of that as there was 12 months ago.

Gordon Cooper came over to see me last Saturday, he does not look a bit well — has got very thin, he told me all about the various boys over there. He had not seen Tonie but heard he was very fit. Holt is nearly the colour of a nigger — you should see some of the boys when they come over first, but they lose it after a few days in bed, or we get used to them. We have such crowds of dysentery cases, the Hospitals are full of very bad cases — also enteric tho that is not so bad in comparison. We also have heaps of jaundice & measles.

Gordon Cooper, from Inverell in northern New South Wales, was another of the young jackaroos that Narrelle knew from back home. And he was like so many of the Anzacs. Aged 21, he was 6 foot tall, weighed a solid 13 stone, had a fair complexion, blue eyes and light brown hair, Gordon enlisted in the 1st ALH on 27 August 1914. He fought on Gallipoli and later spent the rest of his war service in the Middle East. Apart from being thrown off his horse and sustaining concussion and a few cuts and bruises, he managed to survive the war relatively unscathed. However, when Narrelle and Gordon met up in October 1915 he was suffering from influenza. He had been evacuated from Gallipoli on 23 September, and in Malta was sent to St Paul's Hospital. He was then transferred to the large tented convalescent camp at Ghain Tuffieha where he spent six weeks recuperating before returning to Gallipoli.

Among the scandals of Gallipoli, and there were many, were the appalling conditions on the peninsula and the rampant sickness that engulfed the troops. Poor preparations, lack of both medical equipment and suitable staff, and a lack of clear directions and chain of command were all issues that accentuated the medical problems. Furthermore, the British controlled all evacuation processes and medical infrastructure, and as a result Australian authorities had little control over their own

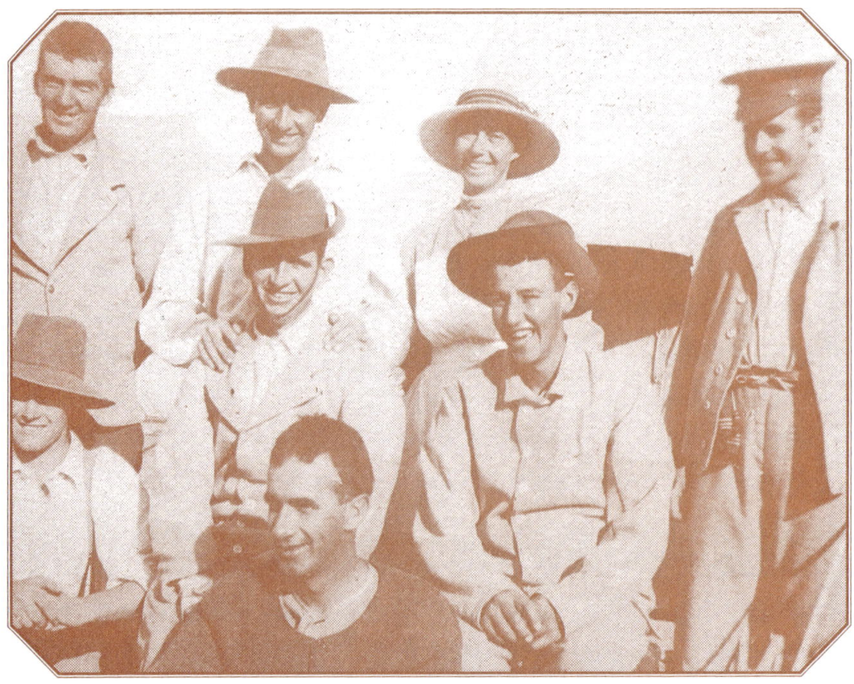

Narrelle and 'her boys', a group of patients at St David's, 1915. (*Hobbes Collection*)

casualties. The rate of disease and sickness, especially in the hot summer months with enteric fever, dysentery and diarrhoea, became hugely costly. Shortages of suitable drinking water and inadequate food supplies simply compounded the health problems for all soldiers on Gallipoli. As a nurse, Narrelle had to deal with the fallout, as she described in her inimitable humorous style.

> *Darlings, I simply have no news for you today, have had a most <u>stodgy</u> fortnight & am getting brain fag with asking the same old patients the same old question. You know we've got practically nothing but Dysentery cases & the one question is 'How often have your bowels acted in the last 24 hrs?' You go round 16 patients in 34 tents & <u>always</u> that is the chief topic of conversation till pon my word when I meet anyone I instinctively say 'How are your bowels etc' — we all say the same, even the M.O.s have said they feel just the same when they go out.*

By late November the weather had changed. Whilst the heat of summer and the dreaded sirocco had gone, it was replaced with cold and rain. Ordinarily this might have been a relief, but in a tent hospital it created chaos.

> *We've had a tremendous change in the climate in the last three days, or the last week really, the cold is tremendous. You could not have imagined it could get so cold in so short a time, it's really very much like the Australian climate. Anyway I'm jolly glad I brought out some thick singlets, my woollie gaiters and fur rug, and my warm nighties. The English sisters mostly didn't bring anything with them, thinking it never got cold here, sillies!*
>
> *Last Sunday night we had a most awful storm — you simply have no idea what it was like, the rain simply fell down in sheets. The poor night nurses crawled off in the morning looking like something the sea had washed up. When we went on, the awful scene that met our gaze, tents blown in, tents down, oh those tents, oh good gracious, I'll never forget them or the sight inside the tents, oh good gracious, nearly every bed was wet, some of them fairly soaked, and we had to get one bed fixed up and lift a patient from a wet bed to a dry one, you know we simply couldn't help laughing at it, it was too funny for words. Since then the cold has been wonderful, it's such a pleasure after the awful heat, but I can hardly hold my pencil to-day, my hands are quite stiff with it.*

Narrelle did not have to put up with running a rain-soaked tent hospital for much longer. After six months' continuous service on Malta at the Valletta Military Hospital and then St David's, she was directed to pack her belongings. Narrelle was being transferred to Sicily.

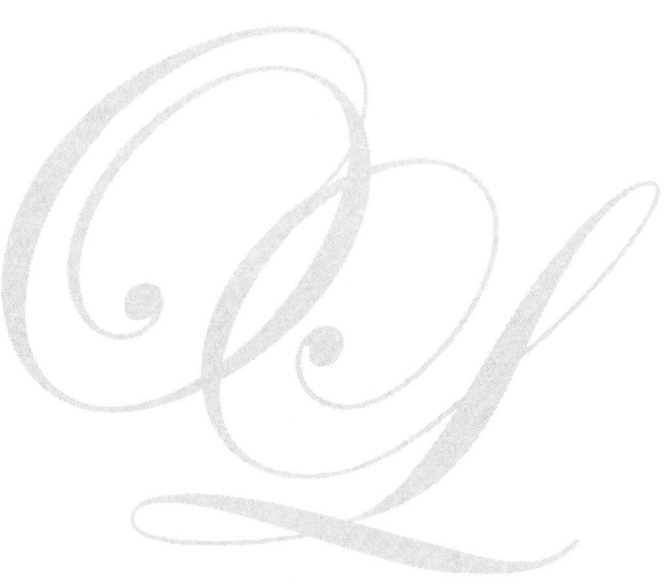

SICILY

Chapter 5

'Thank God I'm Australian'

Sicily, that large, cragged, triangular island at the foot of Italy, halfway between Europe and the African continent, became a base for British wounded from Gallipoli during World War I soon after Italy entered the war on the side of the British and her allies in 1915. Rather than send all convalescent soldiers back to 'Blighty', or England — which involved a dangerous trip across the Mediterranean, through the Straits of Gibraltar and up the French Atlantic coast — or even to Rome, it was decided to use Sicily as a base for a convalescent hospital for officers. Too many ships, both hospital ships and other general merchant navy vessels, had fallen prey to German submarines lurking in the Mediterranean. The heavy loss of life could be minimised by sending 'home' only the most seriously wounded who required specialist medical care and long-term recuperation, or those who would not be taking any further part in the war due to their horrific injuries. The rest would be sent to convalescent hospitals. But these, generally established in refurbished hotels or grand houses and chateaux donated by patriotic individuals, required trained medical staff. So Narrelle, by now a veteran of wartime nursing with six months' continuous service in Malta under her belt, was seconded to the Excelsior Palace Hotel, Palermo, Sicily, along with recently arrived fresh-faced QAIMNS nurses and Red Cross VADs.

Narrelle found Sicily *a strange country*. She came to love it, as she had Malta, and she really tried to immerse herself in the culture by learning Italian, befriending local Sicilian families, and taking every opportunity to visit the amazing historical and ecological sights on the island. But after six months of active service, with precious little relief from the pounding responsibility of wartime nursing, Narrelle's sense of humour was wearing thin. And she was desperately lonely.

Constant travelling can have its ups and downs. Being out of one's comfort zone far from family and friends for any length of time can be difficult. A woman travelling on her own, too, has special problems. It is easy to identify with, and understand, Narrelle's feelings of loneliness and alienation. But if you're on 'active service' and officially part of a British nursing service, working during a war as Narrelle was, then the challenges can be even greater, the stress levels higher, and the responsibilities almost overwhelming.

Narrelle was also separated from her Australian friends, nurses Elsie Welman and Rose Kirkaldie, whom she had met on the boat to London and who were with her on Malta. They managed to stay together and were transferred to a hospital ship, and later to the western front. Narrelle never saw them again. She, on the other hand, was transferred to the Excelsior Palace Hotel in Palermo, and knew only one other British sister from St David's. In Sicily, away from her Australian patients and Australian workmates, Narrelle more than ever felt the full force of, as she saw it, the unreasonably restrictive nature of the British military medical system.

She also felt an increasing sense of powerless to overcome her isolation and homesickness. Whilst Narrelle, an outwardly strong and independent woman, had lived away from her family for some time, she was always within a 'cooee's' distance of them. Even with the isolation of her Brewarrina posting, she had her sister Jean close by at 'Weilmoringle', and many other friends in the district. But it was Narrelle's growing sense of innate difference from the British, and a corresponding belief in herself as an Australian — as a distinct identity — that became increasingly evident during this period of her war service.

By the time Narrelle reached Sicily, she was also beginning to understand exactly what being on active service with the QAIMNS really meant. It finally dawned on her what being part of a British nursing outfit instead of an Australian one entailed. It meant that she was at the mercy of the British, living and working with people very different to her; people with whom she had, she thought, little in common. There was also no guarantee that she would continue to nurse Australian soldiers. Resignation, however, was out of the question. There was still a great need for experienced nurses, and, most importantly, Narrelle was a patriot. Her duty was to remain where she was, with the QAIMNS, even though it became increasingly clear to her that she had made an awful mistake in rushing off to England and not waiting for an opportunity to enlist in the AANS.

WHEN NARRELLE TRANSFERRED TO SICILY IN LATE NOVEMBER 1915, SHE was not to know that plans for the evacuation of Gallipoli were well underway. With winter setting in, the already unbearable conditions on the peninsula were worsening. As Narrelle wrote home, *the tales of frostbite, from the Dardanelles & Salonika, are heartbreaking & I'm so afraid for our dear boys. It seems so impossible that they should all get through safely, & so many of them are having limbs & fingers or whole hands amputated from the result of frostbite. Oh the poor dears, poor dears, be they English or Australian.*

Once the evacuation had taken place, there was much gossip about where the Australian troops would be sent next. Narrelle desperately wanted to get across to her precious Aussie boys in Cairo and Alexandria, and therefore believed that it would be better to remain in the region, rather than request a transfer to England. She was not to know, of course, what would unfold in 1916 in France and Belgium and the role that the Anzacs would play there.

So, alone and lonely, far away from her support base on the other side of the world, and her surrogate family of Australian soldiers, Narrelle developed a strong British–Australian antipathy. She was cross that she was given little notice to move to Sicily in order to nurse English officers.

Well, I cursed again, long & loudly … for I didn't want to come … I realized that I was leaving all the friends I had made over here & all my Australian boys for they wont send them over here … it's worse than being in a private Hospital, and there was so much to be done over there, so much real work … But more than anything I wanted to be with my dear brave Australians, the men I'm so proud of, they have just about 10 times as much spirit as the others.

Narrelle's only release was to pour out her frustrations and feelings in her letters home, which she did regularly, largely with humour and wit, but sometimes with anger and a dose of irritation. In her first letter from Sicily, dated 13 December 1915, Narrelle wrote,

My beloved Peoples,

Well here I am once more in a strange country, feeling somewhat of an outcast, truly a stranger in a stranger's country. It's something quite utterly different to anything I have ever imagined I should be doing. I hardly know where to begin, but I'm going to begin by saying it was the saddest day I've had for a long time, the day I left dear dirty, noisy, adorable Malta …

Today Sicily has been wrapped in cloud & rain, & falling leaves, oh but how I could love it if I was not a machine, or had someone to enthuse with me, instead of people who say, when I am standing awed by the magnificent grandure, the exquisite beauty of Etna, rising up from the hills around, 11,000 feet towards heaven, with its glorious snowcap & purple shades, deepening towards the base to different shades of green. Such exquisite, undreamed of colours, with the clear blue of the Mediterranean on the other side, & I was thinking of the wonderful glory of it all, as the last rays of the sinking sun caught the different peaks & turned them to brown & purple of most exquisite shade & a voice beside me said in a casual way 'Isn't Etna pretty'. Ye gods, oh ye gods that such women should be allowed to gaze on such sights, I could have slain her on the spot & wept, & that is the spirit which dominates this whole outfit.

Thank God I'm Australian. I've said that to myself over & over again, grasping firmly my little Australian badge which never leaves me. But there these English are a strange people, & I shall never understand them nor will they ever understand the Australians.

Narrelle and the medical team sailed from Malta to Syracuse, on the eastern side of Sicily, aboard Lord Dunraven's steam yacht, *Grianaig*. Aged over 70 years old, the Irish peer and avid sailor, who twice tried to win the America's Cup in 1893 and 1895, had donated his large yacht as a hospital ship, and his services as its captain. The *Grianaig* was painted white and had a large red strip all around — a *Crosse Rossa* — to ensure the safety of the medical staff and, with luck, deter the lurking German submarines. The large seas made for a rough and slow journey that took almost nine hours. Arriving at Syracuse at 4.30 in the afternoon, it took time to disembark and get to their hotel, where a tasty meal was served. It was Narrelle's first encounter with Sicilian food and she loved it. Dinner consisted of fish, vegetables and '*principally cauliflower done with much butter, pepper & salt & mashed well, like well mashed potatoes, it was delicious*, as she later related to her family. Narrelle then described her reactions to the Sicilian breakfast served up the following morning.

Went down to breakfast & was regaled with most weird food, three meats on one dish & sliced up lettuce with much oil on it. The meats consisted of tongue that simply rose to heaven, I don't know what made it smell seemed as tho it had died many years ago. Indeed it seemed so ancient that I did not like to think anything so ancient should be tasted by the lips of mere mortals so we side tracked that. Next came ham, well you know over here they do not believe in cooking ham … so we side tracked that, & there was only left some beef which, after the fearfully hard beef at Malta, was simply delicious.

Nurses were restricted in what they were allowed to carry with them on active service. Apart from grumbling earlier in Malta about not having any 'civilian clothes' or being allowed to wear any non-military outfits, Narrelle enumerated in considerable detail her somewhat meagre possessions. These descriptions provide a glimpse of the working wartime nurse, moving from post to post, often with little notice, but with a prescriptive list of essential nursing items. In her first letter from Sicily, she wrote:

We are only allowed 1 trunk (not too big) which as well as our wearing things has to hold a small Kerosene stove, a lantern, iron, any books you have, all sorts of stores in the way of enamel basins, a glass instrument box that Edith sent me, all my instruments (& darlings I've told you in about four different letters what a Godsend those instruments were) & really a thousand & one odds & ends. Then comes my hold-all, goodness only knows what I would do without that hold-all, it carries my boots, aprons, dresses, rugs, old soft rag, cushions & a thousand other things. Then my suit case, heaven alone knows — & my knees — how the lid of that thing closes ever, then my deck chair, it goes everywhere with me, & shall continue to do so — unless it gets worn out in the meantime — till I go back to Australia, in the dim future.

So with all these goods and chattels, Narrelle and the large British medical team boarded the train for the trip around the picturesque eastern coast to Palermo.

At about 11am, we started off on our train journey, through the most glorious scenery possible, skirting all the time along the coast, up past Catania & Messina. The Straights of Messina I loved, so narrow, only about two miles wide with the Italian coast rising up rugged & most beautiful, with little Italian villages tucked away in the mountains, & one thought of all the tales you had ever heard of brigands & all that sort of thing … the new city of Messina, the place they built after the great earthquake [1908] *is a most quaint place, just long low wood huts, row after row of them, & the graves of the poor earthquake victims, or some of them, all in rows along the slope. Made me think of the rows & rows of the graves of our brave lads over in that death trap, Gallipoli.*

Alas, it got dark soon after leaving Messina, & we lost some most wonderful scenery I believe, as we climbed over some mountains & left Etna behind, we skirted around the mountains where Garibaldi tried to cross, & crept into Palermo at about 4am. We were gathered up into a sort of family bus, being followed & stared at by the crowd. We are the first British army people to arrive here within the last 200 years, so are quite pioneers. It's wonderful how little English is spoken here; we will all have to start & learn Italian next.

… It's a most glorious place, quite <u>*the*</u> *hotel of Palermo I should imagine, & has been lent by the management to the British for a Convalescent home for sick Officers…we can take 500 or more if necessary, &, I believe, they are to start arriving on Monday.*

Today, Palermo, the capital of Sicily, is an overcrowded, overdeveloped and decaying city snuggled around a bay that has been compared to Sydney Harbour, sheltered by a mountain range including Monte Pellegrino which holds the shrine of Santa Rosalia, the patron saint of the town. Even in 1915, the small octagonal shaped piazza — Quattro Canti — the centre of old Palermo, with its four elaborate seventeenth-century Spanish Baroque fountains at each corner, was always crowded with overdressed young men looking for trouble or action or both. The clang clang of electric car bells and the rattling of cabs over the cobblestone streets created a sense of the exotic as well as of chaos.

The Excelsior Palace Hotel struggles nowadays to maintain its four-star rating, with its old world charm and faded glory called charming by some, and not such flattering adjectives by others. But when Narrelle was in Palermo, ninety years ago, it was one of the newest and smartest hotels. Constructed in 1891 in the Art Nouveau style for the International Exhibition of Palermo, the Excelsior Palace Hotel was large (Narrelle said over 500 rooms, perhaps a slight exaggeration) but perfect for an officers' convalescent home, with plenty of space to accommodate the medical unit as well.

As the nurses, doctors and orderlies settled in to the Excelsior Palace Hotel, their patients began to arrive. Although they were predominantly English, there were a few Australian officers, but they did little to lift Narrelle's mood. A continuing theme, touched on in Malta but accentuated during her Sicilian stay, was Narrelle's criticism of the military rules, the treatment of nurses, and the British class system in which officers were separated from ordinary soldiers. Notions of a peculiar Australian egalitarianism pervade her reactions to this, which are also tied up with her continued separation anxiety from her 'Australian family' and Australian patients. In her first letter she exploded to her family:

> *Here I am stuck in this rotten Officers Home, where the majority of them, certainly all the Englishmen, think that if you smile at them or stay & talk to them you damn well want to flirt & are longing for them to take notice of you, & we are warned in one of our bally rules that 'Any social intercourse whatever between the Sisters & Medical Officers or the Convalescent Officers or patients is strictly forbidden'. Any infringement of this rule means a military escort back to Malta — I look upon that as my one hope of freedom I assure you — we are not allowed to speak to one of their dear Medical Officers, they must be guarded against our wicked wiles, & yet we are told we need the protection of a man here. We are not to be out after 6pm unless very special permission is granted. We must go out in batches of 2. We must not be absent from a meal without special permission from the C.O. through the Matron. In fact we might just as well be in a convent.*

It was also Christmas time, the first Christmas Narrelle had spent away from her family. It heralded the beginning of a new year, one that would not bring any relief from the war. Indeed, things were only going to get a whole lot worse. Narrelle's obsession to nurse Australian men, her criticism of army rules, the constant irritation provided by her British nursing colleagues, and her strong sense of 'Australianness' formed a constant mantra. Narrelle was always fighting (privately in her correspondence) the British bureaucracy, or the 'powers that be' as she called them, with their 'bally' rules, particularly on nurse fraternisation with officers only, and the strict rules imposed on the nursing staff.

> *I'll go out with some of our nice Australian Officers, but we are not allowed to speak to them outside the building, & scarcely <u>inside</u>. If we do, we are on the look out all the time to see where Matron is, or any of the Medical Officers or Orderlies. Oh I assure you we are leading a strenuous life just now, for as soon as they found I was an Australian they wanted to sort of take possession of me, & naturally I intended talking to them, & do.*

Narrelle described her first war Christmas. She constantly attempted to undermine her superiors with her little acts of 'Australian defiance', as illustrated by the story of the flag in the bread on Christmas Day that she related back to her family, in a letter written on 1 January 1916.

> *We are made to go down the back stairs, used by maids and Orderlies, to our meals, for fear we will stop & speak to the Officers, & we have three separate tables, little ones, just inside the door, & a three flip screen at each table so that we may not be seen, & even on Xmas day we were not allowed to relax from the iron rule for half an hour, not even at meal time … So at dinner that night I just took down my little Australian flag, about 1 and a half by 1 inch in size stuck it in a mound of bread & stuck my little Australian badge on the bread & put it on the table beside my plate … the waiter had to move our screen a bit & the Officers,*

especially the Australian Officers, all saluted it when they saw it, & passed the word round to the others that there was an Australian Sister right there.

They had only been here a few days & they filled up their glasses, & the boy nearest me whispered in a voice, heard only by me 'Australia, we drink your health' & down it went. It was all done in a minute, before Matron could see what was happening. They are dear souls, it's very funny they simply could not stick the rules & regulations in this place.

Narrelle also regularly 'vented her spleen' about her work colleagues to her family. She found them an unimaginative bunch who did not understand her sense of humour, and were totally uninterested in their surroundings. Narrelle's only outlet was to write about her predicament. It was a form of therapy.

Do you know these people in this outfit are <u>the</u> most absolute bores I've ever come across. They simply don't know how to chortle, & most of them simply <u>cannot</u> see the funny side of things. I know they look upon me as a mad Australian, & I don't care, I'm not going to get into their beastly narrow groove ...

How I wish Els was over here to go around and see things with me. It's awful to think of the women who have the chance to see these lovely things & yet who do not appreciate them, & the ones who would love them who cannot come. I would simply <u>love</u> to be able to just wander through Sicily with one or two happy companions. There are some perfectly <u>glorious</u> places, round by Taromina & Siracusa ... just round Palermo there are some perfectly beautiful places, if one could get anyone to go with. But these women have not the soul of hedgehogs. I shall really have to spend some time in England or round about before going back to Australia, to get my bad impression of the English altered. When you girls have been over here, you have just met the charming people, who have laid themselves out to be nice & give you a good time for the few *weeks or days you have been with them, but you come & work among them, & especially in the present day Army ...*

Of course the oranges here are magnificent & the lemons, unfortunately I'm not very fond of oranges, & the flowers, cultivated flowers simply growing wild, oh, it's beautiful, & the misty purple mountains & valleys. If only they were not so cruel to their animals, it spoils the whole thing, the little donkeys nearly make me weep, & the horses, & dogs, for some things I shall be glad to get away. One always has a feeling of 'unsafeness' they are a fierce people ... I laughed at the Major [one of her patients] *this morning. I was standing at the foot of his bed after I had washed him, just talking. Presently he beckoned me over to him & gazed up into my face, after which he said 'Well I've never seen such blue eyes, I've often looked at them & thought they were very blue, but today they are the colour of the sky'. I was talking of Australia & I suppose they turned blue with emotion?!*

IT BECAME APPARENT EARLY IN THE NEW YEAR THAT THE FABULOUS Excelsior Palace Hotel was a white elephant. It was too expensive to run and the volume of patients was low. British generals were spotted in Palermo assessing the situation and the gossip was that the convalescent home would soon be mothballed. With the Gallipoli campaign over, the need for a Sicilian respite centre had passed. Even today there is precious little mention of this British foray in the medical volumes on the war. Staff, including many of the VADs, were transferred back to Malta. Narrelle waited for her turn, but nothing happened. So while she waited for the military to make up their minds, she made the most of her time in Sicily. She was fascinated with the place — its people, culture, scenery and language. Narrelle learnt how to become a traveller, using all her spare time to explore Sicilian sites, and to immerse herself in the Sicilian culture. Because they were not very busy and the work was less demanding, Narrelle began to relax for the first time in six months.

Nurses were generally not given proper leave as soldiers were. There was a general unwritten rule that nurses somehow did not need rest and recreation. Rather, all that nurses required was a 'change of scene', and perhaps 'lighter duties' in order to rest and recuperate. This view was typical across the military. The Australian authorities, for example, at the end of the war, dictated that Australian nurses who required passage back to Australia had to 'work' their way back nursing soldiers or boatloads of wives and children of AIF soldiers who had married during the war. In 1917, Australian nurses were even left out of the original draft repatriation legislation and were hastily inserted during re-drafting. Nurses were also largely ignored under the soldier settlement scheme. Their service was not recognised as equal to that of their brothers, and if a returned nurse married an ex-soldier, she lost her right to apply for a land grant. Discrimination was obvious but nurses were powerless to do anything about it. So, amazingly, Narrelle's transfer to Sicily after six months continuous service in Malta was seen in some quarters as her unofficial 'leave'. However, she took full advantage of her situation and location and set off to see the sights.

From this point on in her war service, Narrelle was not only an Australian nurse but an Australian traveller. As she journeyed to her different postings, she attempted to read novels and books set in the country she was visiting so that she could learn about the history, culture and people of a particular place. She purchased a copy of renowned British travel writer and Victorian Orientalist Norma Lorimer's *On Etna* which she recommended to her family to read as it had *good descriptions of Sicilian life*. *On Etna* is a romance novel set in Sicily at the turn of the century.

Miss Norma Lorimer and her travelling companion Mr Douglas Sladen wrote many travel books and novels, both independently and as co-authors. Their *More Queer Things about Japan* was a bestseller as was their book *Queer Things about Sicily*, first published in 1905. Sladen, founder and editor of *Who's Who*, was a prolific writer, traveller and general bon vivant. Throughout her life (1864–1948), Lorimer travelled extensively to North Africa, Japan, Asia, Canada and Egypt. During the war two films were made based on her book *There was a King in Egypt*, described as a time-travel novel whose leading character 'finds adventure and romance in Ancient Egypt'. In her 1901 travel book, *By the Waters of Sicily*, Lorimer described the Sicilian tourist cycle as follows: 'February is the German season in Sicily, March is the English one, and in April and May America sends over her fair daughters to sample the island and carry away specimens of its antiquities.' Narrelle need not have worried about coming across German tourists. The war had halted the regular tourist trade to the island. But the sites they traditionally yearned to see were still there, such as the fabulous Roman and Greek ruins around Syracuse, especially the fifth-century BC Greek theatre cut out of rock; the Roman amphitheatre, similar to the Colosseum, used centuries before for gladiatorial spectacles; and the amazing twelfth-century cathedral at Monreale, with its stunning gilded interiors.

Narrelle thoroughly explored Palermo, dominated by its wonderful cathedral and multitude of historical sites with their Islamic influences and Gothic styles. She visited the fishing village of Mondello along the coast road, which today is almost an outer suburb of Palermo and favoured for its beaches. As Narrelle described it:

> *Mondello is a dear quaint little fishing village, right on the coast, right round Monte Pellegrino & over shadowed by another mountain, & as far as one could see, were rugged mountains, jutting right into the sea, with the most wonderful purple shades, & soft greys & browns, all melting into one another, & the whole melting away into soft purple mists. If any of you girls come to England again, you must come to Sicily if only for a few days. I love it, the soft grey green of the olive trees & the deep green of the oranges & lemons, with the splash of colour made by the ripe fruit, the almond trees just coming into bud & a perfect carpet of the most exquisite green, with masses & masses of those yellow flowers that close up at night … & the most exquisite purple iris, just little short stems like jonquils. I would like to be here in the spring, I think it will be magnificent.*

Narrelle also had a wonderful trip out to Monreale, *pronounced Mon-ryarlee … It's right up the side of a mountain, most beautiful … I love Monreale best, with its cathedral & quaint streets, prickly pear orchards, olive groves, lemon & orange groves, & best of all its most wonderful views … I'll tell you, & all its legends & points of interest, of course really, I love Sicily …* This small town, inland from Palermo, and surrounded by mountains, is famous for its twelfth-century cathedral, built for the Norman king William II and adorned with gilt mosaics. Blending both Christian and Arab cultural influences, and incorporating the most beautiful Benedictine cloister with 228 columns, this cathedral remains one of the best examples of Norman architecture in Sicily.

While at the Excelsior Palace Hotel, Narrelle experienced an earthquake, a common feature of the region. It was *<u>most</u> weird, this bally hotel shook like billyho. I trust they are not going to make a hobby of it and treat us to them often.* Devastating earthquakes are a part of Sicilian history. Narrelle read and wrote about the earthquake that totally destroyed Messina in December 1908. Up to 100,000 people were killed from the quake and ensuing tidal wave.

In a letter to her nieces, Jean and Barbie, who had been sent to boarding school in Sydney in early 1916, Narrelle painted an enticing picture of Sicily, including her train trip where she passed through the newly rebuilt town of Messina.

> *Palermo is a very beautiful place, not so much the city as the outside places, I've been to several of them and love them, it's all so different to anything I have ever seen. They have crowds of little donkeys, & really, the way they load them up is too dreadful, sometimes you can scarcely see the donkey for the load, numbers of them are not much bigger than a dog, they seem to be able to carry & draw, weights out of all comparison to their size, really they are most wonderful …*
>
> *There are some very wonderful old churches here, and wonderful ruins & places dating back to 1115, I must get you some PCs* [postcards] *of different places. The thing that amuses me are the flocks of goats, driven through the streets, and milked anywhere in the street or on the pavement.*

They are absolutely disgusting really, but no one seems to think anything at all of it, they wander through, and cows, with calves tied to their tails, dozens of them, the goat herd will wander along ahead of this goats calling to them, & calling out 'Latte' which is Italian for milk, in Malta they used to call 'Harleep'. The policemen here wear the most wonderful hats, I have been trying to get a snapshot of them, they also wear long capes below their knees, instead of coats, the soldiers nearly all wear capes too, & they go in for the most gorgeous colours for their uniforms. Of course when they go to the front they leave the colours behind.

… I would love to think that I would come back here again some day when the war is over, & just go all round Sicily. There are two beautiful places over on the Eastern side Syracusa [Syracuse] *& Taromina, the latter is <u>most</u> beautiful they say, we just passed through part of it coming round here. We landed at Syracusa (or Siracusa) & took the train there, round by Catania & Messina, the latter place was destroyed five years ago with a most fearful earthquake.*

Not only did Narrelle spend as much time as she could sight-seeing, she complemented her tourist adventures by learning Italian. She discovered that most Italians and Sicilians spoke some French but very few knew English and that made communication difficult. As she was mainly on night duty at the Excelsior, she thought she would have plenty of time to study. There was little to do in the wee small hours, as she and a VAD only had three patients to care for. But Narrelle found it difficult to learn because the task kept putting her to sleep.

I get so awfully sleepy when I try to study, & when I try to write, I find the pen wandering all over the paper like a spider, it's so beastly for I meant to do so much while on night duty having so much time, but instead I have done less than ever, & have to keep getting up & walking up & down the hall, till I waken up again, then start afresh.

By attempting to learn the language, Narrelle acknowledged that she felt something special for Sicily and its people. She identified with its natural and untamed landscape and could see something of her own personality in the physical countryside. *I love Sicily, it catches hold of one somehow, perhaps it does with me, more than it would to be English, being more a lover of the wild, for it's wild right enough.*

There were also plenty of invitations to various entertainments held by local Sicilian families of note and expats. Narrelle met *a rather nice Sicilian family. Mother, three daughters & son-in-law, two of the girls are rather sweet, one reminds me very much of Kit & I love to watch her trying to speak English, she looks so distressed when she cannot think of a word.* Narrelle played tennis and socialised with them when she was off duty. The family provided her with a semblance of normality from her military existence, and she could practice her halting Italian with them. But these contacts did little to counter her loneliness. Narrelle was incredibly lonely in Sicily. She did not have a special companion or friend amongst the nursing staff. There were no Australians like Elsie and Rose and Narrelle felt she had nothing in common with the English nurses and VADs. They were not interested in looking at the historical sites and Narrelle felt they were socially inferior to her. *They are rather common, and did not like going about to see things, I mean beautiful views, or old churches, or ruins & all that sort of thing.*

Narrelle was particularly embarrassed at being invited to a very swish 'do' and being directed by her Matron to wear a certain outfit that was totally inappropriate for the occasion. This incident revealed something of Narrelle's concept of herself as a refined, middle-class Australian woman who had been brought up in a certain manner and was aware of the codes and etiquette of the British upper classes. This was in contrast to the Matron, the woman in charge of the nursing unit, and her inability (deliberate or not) to 'read' the etiquette codes correctly. The result was that the nurses from the Excelsior were highly embarrassed, or indeed Narrelle was. As her war service continued, this issue of class and the 'types of people' with whom she associated in the QAIMNS was increasingly a problem for her as she lost contact with Australians.

She wrote in a letter dated 12 January 1916:

On Saturday night we were invited to a concert to the Villa Igiea. [Built in 1898, the Grand Hotel Villa Igiea today is one of the most luxurious five-star hotels in Sicily.] *It was a very swagger affair. Countess this & Baroness that, with a Princess or two thrown in. We of course should have been in our Mess Kit — outdoor frock & cap — but no, Matron insisted upon us wearing our hats, & she kept her coat on & a grey muffler round her throat, & lay back in her chair & went to sleep. No more idea of the fitness of things than a mouse. Of course everyone else was in full evening dress & the Sisters & Nurses at the Villa were in their Mess Kit. I was furious, it was like going to a dinner in a blouse & skirt you had worn in the morning, but never mind.*

The Villa is a most beautiful place. It was being built originally by Prince — & funds ran out. I don't wonder, it's a most magnificent building, then it was taken over by some-one else & finished, & turned into a huge Hotel, fitted up like a palace, golf course, tennis courts etc. I must try & get some snap shots of it. [None of these photographs have survived.] *Then a month or two ago a Mr & Mrs Beaumont decided they would like to take part of it for a convalescent home for officers under the Red X. They are very wealthy English but came to Sicily nearly every year. They came out, took one wing of the hotel, with 100 beds in it, brought out 9 Sisters & 9 VADs, have been here a month, just sightseeing, and got their first convalescent Officers on Saturday.*

MEANWHILE NARRELLE'S AUSTRALIAN FRIENDS, BOTH THOSE SHE KNEW from Brewarrina, and others she met whilst nursing on Malta, were all in Egypt, cooling their heels after the evacuation from Gallipoli. She regularly received letters and postcards from a number of them, and then related their news back to her family. When her mother asked about the billies, a fabulous idea whereby voluntary organisations arranged to send all Australian soldiers a Christmas present of a billy can stuffed full of goodies, Narrelle replied that:

> *Yes all the boys got their 'Billies' at Xmas, on Lemnos I think, after the evacuation. I had letters from some of them, telling me about them, & how they felt like kiddies at Xmas, with their stockings, being handed a billy & going off to look & see what was inside it. They really* <u>*are*</u> *like children you know, when they come over from the trenches, the least little thing makes them happy & amuses them.*
>
> *… I had a letter from Stuart Glennie today from Egypt, also from dear Holt & some others. Geoff Yeomans has his commission in the 1st Batt. Holt says Frank is very fat … They are all camped fairly close around. Isn't it nice for them all being together … Poor old Holt said, 'I'm not saying anything about the evacuation, in a way it was a merciful blessing, to get away from it, but it was jolly rotton leaving all one's mates over there. Oh the joy of our first fresh water bath, after having only salt water for seven months. To be able to go & soak in it, real fresh water, & then stay in your bunk all day, just going out for meals'. At the end of Holt's letter he had written 'I very much like the scent of your notepaper'.*

Narrelle's mother had sent her a bunch of boronia which she had locked up with her writing pad, and it scented everything in the suitcase including her notepaper.

Stuart Glennie was from Glen Innes in northern New South Wales, and had only recently arrived in Egypt. The tall, solidly built, 22-year-old station hand enlisted in July 1915. On his enlistment papers Glennie stated that he trained as a cadet whilst at school at Barker College. On arrival in Egypt he transferred as a gunner to the 14th Field Artillery Battery. Narrelle never caught up with Stuart Glennie as he was transferred to France in June 1916 and was killed in action on 30 September 1917.

Narrelle was also in regular contact with Frank Webb, the overseer from 'Weilmoringle', who had joined up with friend and fellow jackaroo Jim Langwell in September 1915. They enlisted together, Frank as a driver and Jim as a gunner in the 2nd Ammunition Column, 4th Field Artillery Brigade, and embarked from Melbourne on 16 November. Frank's father, William Webb, was an inspector of railways and, in his youth, the family had moved around New South Wales. After school, Frank worked at 'Gunyerwarildi' for his uncle, Donald MacKay (married to Kit, Narrelle's sister), and from 1910 he worked at 'Weilmoringle' for George Magill (married to Jean, another of Narrelle's sisters). Frank Webb, or 'Franks' as Narrelle referred to him, became one of her regular correspondents.

> *Had a letter from Frank last night, he is a quaint soul, really, his remarks re Cairo are too funny, I wonder what he would say to this place, it's the one blot on Palermo, but those boys have lived such clean, healthy lives, that's why Holt* [Hardy] *and Tonie* [Hordern] *were able to go through all those months and look well at the end of it. Frank said 're Cairo, the place disgusts me, I'd like to burn more than half of it down, give me the free healthy life of the bush with my horse and dog, and a chap doesn't want anything more than to lead a clean healthy busy life, and I don't care how soon I get back to it'. He thinks Jim has altered very much, or else he has got to know him better. (I know it's the close comradeship of camp life, the clinging to the one person who has the same interests, the same home, when away in a foreign country at a time like this.)*

Narrelle felt that she could interpret the soldiers' experiences to those back home because they were all on active service on the other side of the world. She continued to gently 'lecture' her family about the virtues of the Australian men. In a letter to her impressionable nieces away at boarding school, she wrote:

> *Kiddies, you must be very very proud of our Australian men. They are simply splendid, not only in their work, but in their sufferings. Do all you can to help get them with comforts, & write Franks & Jack, & Jim Langwell as often as you can. Remember that they may never return, & it is the greatest joy they have, over here, hearing from the home people,*

& oh <u>how</u> they look forward to letters. Only we, who have been over here & seen their dear faces light up when they get a letter, or how sad they look when someone else gets a letter & they do not. I write <u>ever</u> so many Australians, simply because I've seen that look.

NARRELLE'S BLINDING LOVE FOR HER AUSTRALIAN 'BOYS', AND HER increasingly negative view of the British, led her to make decisions that would adversely impact on her future. In early 1916, all staff at the Excelsior were offered up to six weeks' leave due to the lack of work. Narrelle could have gone back to England — as Rose and Elsie did — taken leave, and then waited for a posting to France. But Narrelle was blinded by her prejudices and the only direction she wanted to go was East, to Egypt, because that was where the Australians were currently based. Although there were rumours flying around about possible destinations for the Australian troops, it took some time for the news to reach Sicily that the Anzacs were going to France, with only the Australian Light Horse to remain behind in Palestine.

The Excelsior Palace was wound up in March 1916, with over 200 nursing sisters transferred back to England. The Malta operation was to be scaled back as well. Clearly Narrelle did not know where she was to go next or what the military had in store for her. With no clear strategy herself and no special friend to team up with, she expected to return to Malta to take her six weeks' leave. Narrelle seemed resigned to the transient nature of wartime nursing. As she explained to her family:

... in the Army you never know from day to day where you will be, & you come across people, make friends of them & suddenly one day you find they have been yanked away, or you have, & you never see them again, & quite often you never ever hear of them again, unless you have agreed to write, & then these days one never has much time for writing any but <u>old</u> friends, & so they pass on.

Narrelle was not going to leave Sicily, however, without one last great tourist adventure. In her last days in Palermo, before returning to Malta, Narrelle went on a climbing expedition to Monte Cuccio, one of the highest mountains near Palermo. She described the outing in great detail to her family. The party included two doctors, Major Bardswell and Colonel Thomas Percy Legg; the Bartrams, a mother and daughter team; Narrelle; and Nurse Williams, her night nursing sister companion. Narrelle knew Thomas Legg reasonably well for he was originally posted to Malta, and was with her at St David's. An unmarried Harley Street surgeon from London in his early forties, Narrelle was to see more of Colonel Legg in the future. Although Narrelle was on night duty and had had little sleep, she was ready for the adventure. After breakfast and a change of clothes, as Narrelle related to her family:

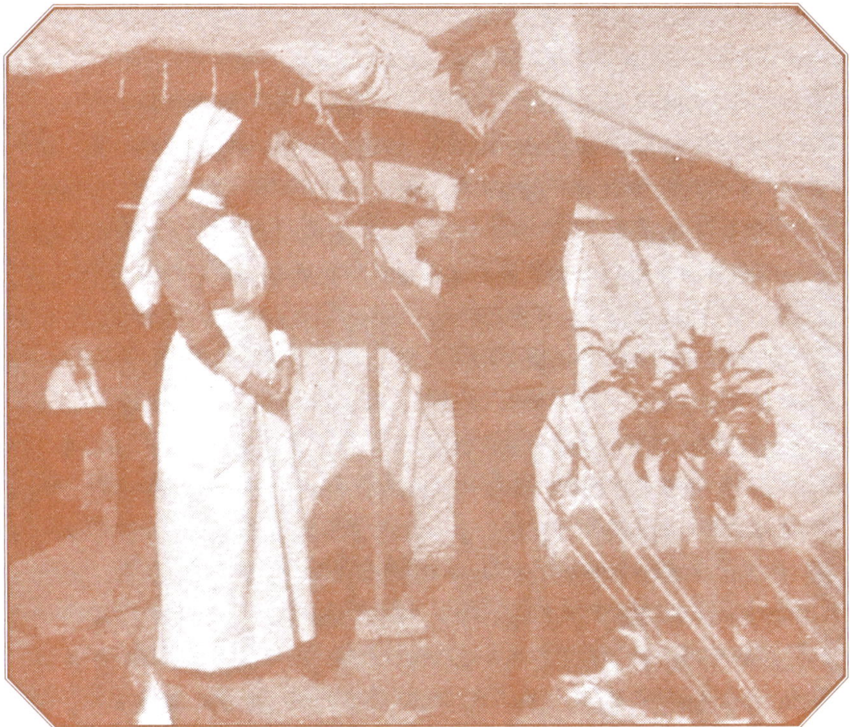

Colonel Thomas Legg, a friend of Narrelle, who served in Malta, Sicily and Mesopotamia, at St David's, 1915. (*Hobbes Collection*)

[I] *got the waiter to put up our lunch — hard boiled eggs, sardines, fresh rolls, cheese, fruit & bottle of wine, to be carried to the top by our guide, well that's the last I saw of it but there by hangs a tale — Major Bardwell, Col Legg, Nurse & I went in one carriage & the Bartrams in another, & we drove to a little village called Boccadifilo (an old Arab village), we left the carriages there & Mrs Bartram mounted a mule with the tucker bags & our coats, & we all started to walk, miles round the foot of the mountain to get round the side of it, I had my Kodak slung on my back & got some ripping snaps, if they turn out right* [none of these photographs have survived].

Col Legg & I decided we would not rush things at first, but get to the top by easy stages, ahem — we did, at least we never got to the top, they told us there was a track all the way up, that damn track never met our eye till we were half way down again — to continue, from the time we left the road winding around the base of the mt up a glorious valley it was one climb at times on our hands & knees, positively, I've never in all my life met anything like it, but oh the glorious beauty of it all, I shall never never forget it, & I simply cannot describe the sight as we got higher & higher, the 7 of us were scattered over the face of that mountain — devoid of trees — like goats, each one trying to make their own track.

Poor little Col Legg was getting most desperately tired, & as for me, well there were moments when I simply lay on the face of the mountain & panted, we clung to tussocks with one hand & clawed on our side like crabs, for a few hundred feet then we would sit down & gaze out over the mountains, away below us was a wee molehill that had looked a fair sized mount when we were under it, & oh, oh that glorious soft purple mist & the great sharp peaked rugged chains of mountains one behind the other, & away in the distance snow capped Etna, & away down the most wonderful valley — Conca d'Ora — & where-ever you looked, the most wonderful colouring, from the wild flowers, such flowers, I nearly wept with sheer joy at it all, but upwards, once more we had to go on, Col. Legg stopping every now & again to say 'Sister I'm not going any further, I absolutely refuse', 'Gosh don't let Mrs Bartram beat you to the *top' & once more the little man would come on. He really <u>was</u> looking very tired, & as for me, I could have lain down in my own tracks cheerfully, & oh the <u>heat</u>.*

At last, I was about 20 feet above Col, when suddenly he gave a loud exclamation & dropped to the ground, 'damn I've twisted my knee' he said. I wasn't a bit sympathetic for a moment, for I didn't believe him — nor did anyone else afterwards — but when I saw him getting a bit white & beads of perspiration rolling off him, I clambered down to him, I was afraid the poor little beggar was going to faint, & simply did not know what to do, we were about 200 feet from the top, & the very worst pinch to go up, all the others were at the top & could not see or hear us & the mule & man were half way down the side of the mountain & the man could not speak a word of English, & it was 1.30, well of course I felt an awful beast for having urged the poor little soul to go on. Well, we waited for a bit, hadn't even any stuff to bandage his knee with, so we just rested, then we decided we were decidedly hungry & thirsty, so Col rooted in his bag, knapsack — & found a bottle of mineral water, two rolls & two oranges, & a piece of cheese that had melted with the heat.

Well after we had emptied the knapsack or haversack, we thought we had better try and get down to the mule, before the knee began to swell & get stiff. Do you know even then I had my doubts as to the genuineness of that twist, but when we came to slopes where it was impossible to walk, he would sit down on the ground & slither along, <u>over most awful thistles</u>, so I decided no human being would <u>wellfully</u> [sic] *slide over those thistles for fun & that he really <u>must</u> have hurt his knee.*

I wanted him to ride the donkey when we got to it. He said he never could sit on a horse when it was walking over smooth ground & was certain he could not stick on a donkey going down that mountain, & just as I started to tell him it was quite easy & would be much better for his knee, the donkey sat down hurridly, three times in succession where upon he turned upon me & said 'Yes, I know what <u>you</u> want Sister, you want to see me repeat Major Harding's friends progress down the mountain, when he only touched ground twice all the way down'. I certainly must *admit I wouldn't have got on that donkey if I'd had to crawl the whole way down. Some time after we started to descend the others missed us & crawled round the top to see what was the matter, we could not make them hear, but they guessed what had happened when they saw Col slithering down the side.*

I was awfully disappointed not to get right to the top, but I couldn't leave the poor little beggar, so we went down instead, & then waited half way down the mountain side till the others came. They simply would not believe us, & to this day jeer at us when we mention Monte Cuccio. We did not get back till 7.15 pm, all dog tired but happy having been up a mountain that few Sicilians have tried to climb.

Narrelle's Italian sojourn was at an end. She was finally ordered back to Malta. The following week she packed her bags, caught the train back along the coast to Syracuse, and sailed the short distance to Malta.

India

Chapter 6

'DAMNED MOIST AND UNCOMFORTABLE'

NARRELLE ARRIVED BACK IN MALTA AT THE END OF MARCH 1916. IT WAS spring, a perfect time to be on the island. But Malta was like a ghost town compared to the chaos and activity of the past year. Whilst there were still patients on the island, there was precious little work to do for the hundreds of nursing staff. With the evacuation of Gallipoli in December 1915, the need for Malta's medical facilities had diminished. At the start of 1916, there were 334 medical officers, 913 nurses and 2032 other members of the RAMC on Malta. By mid year, the medical staff was halved, and only about 400 nurses remained. This hiatus was not to last long, with an influx of wounded and ill soldiers from the Salonika campaign (fought in Macedonia against the Turks and Bulgarians) that began in summer and autumn 1916.

In the meantime, nurses and medical staff were off duty, hanging around waiting for notification of their next posting. Most believed it was just a question of time before they headed back to England, and possibly France. Shifts in the direction of the war, the slow machinations of command decisions from the War Office back in London, and inadequate shipping were largely behind the delays. Lists for England were regularly posted and eagerly scanned by all, but Narrelle's name did not appear. Matron Hoadley, in charge of nursing staff on Malta, liked Narrelle and wanted to keep her there for as long as possible. Narrelle knew that and hoped that if she had to stay that she might again be posted to St David's which was still operating, with about 400 patients, albeit few of them Australians. With plenty of time on her hands, Narrelle went out and visited the hospital that was once her second home. She reminisced about her time there, and how in the spring it looked beautiful with the gardens in full bloom, *simply a blaze of colour, & all the paths picked out in white stones.*

But once again Narrelle felt a deep loneliness. She missed her friends. And she was still cross about the restricted fraternisation rules, which she firmly blamed on the 'loose' English women. As she related to her family:

> *It's so strange here without Rose & Elsie, I keep turning off to go to their old room, & then remember they are not here. There are none of my friends here now, it's rather lonely, little Trumble & Beattie & Gibbie are still out at St David's, but it's such a decidedly long way out there, & you have no chance finding them out as we cannot telephone. Malta is beastly now really, the blessed V.A.D. & some of the Sisters have spoilt the whole Island. They acted like fools, and only came out here to have a jolly good time, consequently they have brought out the same rules pretty well that we had in Palermo. It's perfectly disgusting, these women simply cannot help themselves, they are man mad. Consequently if we are seen speaking to one now there is the very dickens of a row.*

One of the highlights of her return to Malta was a huge pile of letters. Over 42 letters were waiting for her from various family members, as well as letters and postcards from Holt Hardy, Frank Webb and all the boys, so she heard the latest news that many were off to France, which now meant, of course, further away from her.

WHILE NARRELLE WAS MARKING TIME IN MALTA, THERE WERE developments in the war on a largely unknown front. Called the Mesopotamian campaign, it does not generally feature in histories of World War I, for reasons that will become apparent shortly. But it had a profound impact on Narrelle. The Mesopotamian campaign fought against the Turks in what we now call Iraq has not received the same interest and coverage as other theatres of war. Indeed, it may come as a surprise to some to learn that there was fighting going on in that region at all. So what exactly were the British doing in Mesopotamia?

In the lead up to World War I, significant changes occurred within the British Navy, arguably the finest in the world at that time. One of the changes involved how warships were powered. With the discovery of commercial quantities of oil in Persia (now Iran) in 1908, and the creation of the Anglo–Persian Oil Company in 1909, there was a shift from coal-fired ships to oil. In 1913, the British government, under instructions from Winston Churchill and the British Navy, partly nationalised the company in order to secure oil supplies. With the war underway a year later, the British were keen to make sure that their supplies of oil were safe. They wanted to protect Abadan, a small island in the Shatt-el-Arab, the vast waterway that links the mighty Tigris River with the Persian Gulf between Mesopotamia and Persia, and the pipeline to vital oilfields in Persia.

Mesopotamia was part of the Ottoman Empire, so when the Turks came into the war on the side of Germany in late 1914, British forces from India, under the Indian Expeditionary Force, moved into the Shatt-el-Arab to protect their interests. But instead of merely securing a presence in the Tigris Delta and stopping at Abadan, the British continued on. They captured Basra, a key city on the Tigris River with a population of about 60,000, with relative ease as the smallish Turkish forces retreated north.

Buoyed by this success, the campaign, run from Simla in India with limited input from the War Office in London, was continued with the ambitious view of going all the way to Baghdad. The vast majority

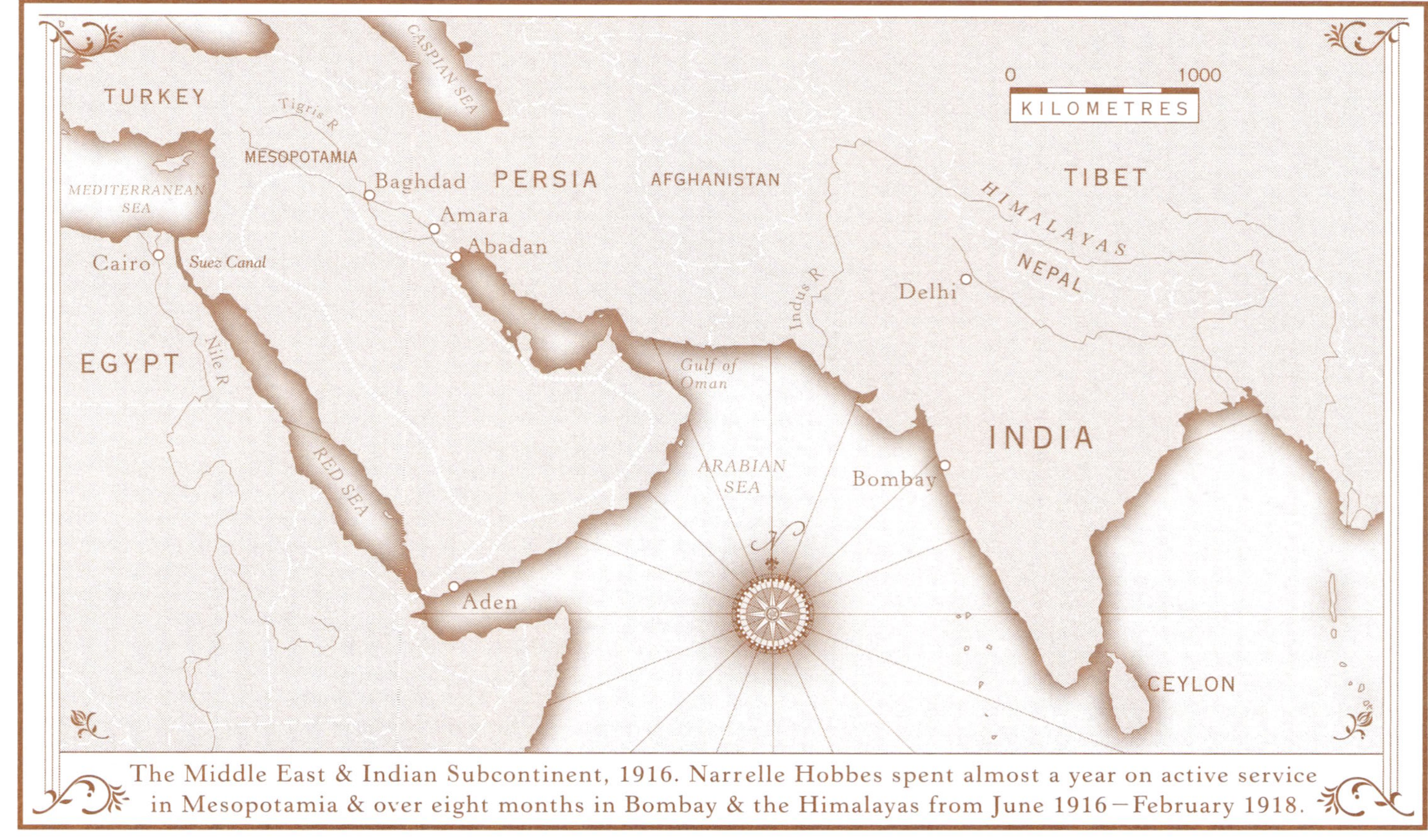

The Middle East & Indian Subcontinent, 1916. Narrelle Hobbes spent almost a year on active service in Mesopotamia & over eight months in Bombay & the Himalayas from June 1916 – February 1918.

of the Indian Expeditionary Force was, at this point, made up of native Indian soldiers. Through early 1915, the British moved 90 miles (144 kilometres) up the Tigris to Amara, and then on to Kut, a further 150 miles (240 kilometres) upstream, encountering little resistance or opposition from the Turkish defenders. Instead of staying put in Kut, the British leader of the expedition, General Charles Townshend, continued on towards Baghdad despite being underresourced and with lines of communication stretched precariously thin. The unforgiving climate also took a heavy toll on his soldiers. The Indian Expeditionary Force came within 30 miles (48 kilometres) of Baghdad when the Turks, led by German Baron von der Goltz, commander-in-chief of Turkish forces in Mesopotamia, mounted a battle at Ctesiphon. Outmanoeuvred and overpowered, Townshend and his men retreated back down the Tigris to Kut. Encircled by Turkish forces, the British held out for 147 days, but reinforcements failed to arrive. In late April 1916, General Townshend and his 11,800 strong garrison surrendered to the Turks. It was an ignominious defeat and the end of a flawed and badly planned campaign.

Hot on the heels of the Gallipoli debacle, the fall of Kut was seen as one of the worst British military disasters of the war, severely damaging the prestige of the British Army. It was the second defeat at the hands of the Turks (with assistance from German generals) in four months. It was a low, low point. Within a few months the British public were aghast and appalled as details of the distant Mesopotamian campaign leaked out into the press. Captured British soldiers were brutally treated by their captors as they made the long trek northwards to POW camps in Anatolia, Turkey. Over 4200 men, or one-third of the total number of captured soldiers, died on the way.

Not only was the whole campaign a haphazard jumble of egos, military incompetence and unrealistic expectations, but the physical, geographical and medical problems encountered by the British forces in Mesopotamia were extraordinary. The overstretched communication links, combined with inadequate transportation and medical facilities contributed to the debacle. Stories emerged about the aftermath of the

Battle of Ctesiphon, in which the treatment of wounded and ill Indian and British soldiers beggars belief. A major in charge of one of the hospital ships, the *Varela* at Basra, described the arrival of the *Medjidieh*, part of a river convoy that had been ten days on the Tigris River with minimal medical staff in attendance. From a distance, the boat looked as if it was …

> *… festooned with ropes. The stench when she was close was quite definite, and I found that what I mistook for ropes were dried stagactites* [sic] *of human faeces … a certain number of men were standing and kneeling on the immediate perimeter of the ship. Then we found a mass of men huddled up anyhow — some with blankets and some without. They were lying in a pool of dysentery about 30 feet square. They were covered with dysentery and dejecta generally from head to foot. With regard to the first man I examined, I put my hand into his trousers, and I thought that he had a haemorrhage. His trousers were full almost to his waist with something warm and slimy. I took my hand out, and thought it was a blood clot. It was dysentery.*

The lack of adequate medical treatment for soldiers of the British army was reminiscent of days long past. It was a disgrace.

The medical assistance for the campaign was controlled by the Indian government through Army Headquarters at Simla, the stretched and underresourced Indian Medical Service, and the No 3 British General Hospital which, from November 1915, was based at Basra. Whilst the full extent of the medical and transport problems was not identified until a Royal Commission reported in 1917, it was clear before the fall of Kut that urgent action, especially on the medical front, was required. The conclusion of the Gallipoli campaign, as we have seen, freed up medical staff and equipment in Malta and Egypt. The 23rd Stationary Hospital and the 32nd British General Hospital, without nursing sisters, was immediately transferred to Mesopotamia, embarking from Egypt in March 1916.

The hospital ship *Assaye* later transported 28 British nursing sisters under the supervision of Matron Hodgins arriving in Kuwait on 1 April. They were part of the 23rd Stationary Hospital, and one of the first groups of QAIMNS to be sent to Mesopotamia by the British authorities. It took a week for all the supplies and medical equipment to be transferred on to a smaller boat, the *Aronda*, which could safely cross the bar and enter the shallower waters of the Shatt-el-Arab. During a violent storm, some of the precious medical equipment ended up in the water. Eleven of the nursing sisters were allocated to hospital ship duties, mainly travelling to and from Bombay, eight were sent to the No 3 British General Hospital in Basra, and the remainder were sent on to Amara. A new broom, in the form of Surgeon General F. H. Treherne and his offsider Colonel Fell from the RAMC, arrived in early May 1916 to transform the medical, communication and transportation services in Mesopotamia.

NARRELLE'S NEXT POSTING WAS PART OF THESE MAJOR MEDICAL reforms. On Saturday 15 May 1916, exactly a year to the day that she left London for Malta, Narrelle boarded the hospital ship *Marama*, staffed by New Zealand nurses: *the N.Z. Sisters were pets, I simply loved getting among them, they are so different to the others, dear souls, & the Matron was charming.* Narrelle left Malta for the last time, heading towards Alexandria and India. She was posted to the 22nd Stationary Hospital, Indian Expeditionary Force. She was, as Narrelle called it, on her way to 'Meso'.

The voyage took three days. On Tuesday 18 May, the group arrived in Alexandria, and were accommodated at the Khedinial Hotel, once *the Hotel of Alex*, which had been turned into a nurses' home during the war. According to Narrelle it was a *seething mass of women*. For the next ten days, Narrelle again played the tourist. She certainly made the most of the visit and took every opportunity to see the sights. But Narrelle did not like Alexandria, or Alex, as she described in a letter to her family.

Alex, well yes Alex was some place, but I wouldn't like to live there. It's not a typically Egyptian town, & with the exception of Pomey's Pillar & its old Catacombs has little attraction for visitors. The town is almost entirely Italian in character, & is peopled by so many different races that it hardly seems Egypt at all. Ras-el-tin fort is rather an attraction & Monzah gardens are beautiful the wonderful, brilliant colourings of the flowers, the rich growth of trees & shrubs, & the palm trees, I loved the gardens, & then outside the gardens, running out into the desert was the Mohomoudi canal, a perfectly charming place. Miss Stow [a nursing friend] *& I walked for miles along it one day taking snap shots … the 'STINK' of 'Alex' was atrocious, absolutely, it was a dirty place. We used to think Malta was dirty but dear life in Malta was clean to Alex.*

Narrelle also made a trip to Cairo. She had heard so much about Cairo from the boys, both good and bad, and she wanted to experience it first hand. It was a three-hour train trip from Alex to Cairo, and they stayed overnight. She enjoyed exploring Cairo, the pyramids, riding camels, and the bazaars. Narrelle loved being the tourist. As she wrote home in a letter dated 21 May 1916:

Alexandria is a beastly place altogether, but Cairo, a dream. Some of us were given 24 hours leave so we flew up there, it only took three hours from here, it was wonderful, & the colouring & sights, all along the line, up the Nile Valley is exactly like the old prints one used to gaze upon in one's infancy, Ruth in the fields of Boaz etc, really the colours one sees in pictures of Egypt is not a bit exaggerated as a rule, & the quaint old water wheel worked by a bullock going round in a circle & the wheat is thrashed by a bullock or two wandering round & round in a ring, dragging a sort of sledge over the wheat.

… The valley of the Nile reminded me just exactly of the plains [near Brewarrina], *only covered with thousands of patches of green stuff & yellow wheat & corn, with funny humpy buffaloes tethered, just able to feed the length of the rope, men & women in long flowing garments of*

many hues, reaping & gathering the bundles of wheat, loading donkeys & camels with it, & with green stuff, & every here & there a quaint old wheel for drawing water, being worked by two oxen, & in another place where all the wheat was being carried & placed in heaps, two oxen were harnessed to a sort of sledge — if the harvest was a big one, if small one animal simply dragged along a log of wood — & dragged it round & round in one spot over the wheat to thresh it, & then we saw the mounds of grain after all the straw had been lifted away, & it was being put through a sieve … & then at the end of the day, they all started off back to the quaintest little mud villages, quite impossible to describe, some surrounded by palm trees. I managed to get a snap shot of one, but do not know how it will turn out, as the train was just moving slowly down at a station.

We went to the Continental Hotel, an awfully nice place. Shepherds [the famous hotel in Cairo] *is too rapid, & expensive but this was an awfully nice place. We just got in in time for dinner, then we went for a drive to the Nile & round by Ghizerah & the garden city. If it had been moonlight we would have gone straight out to the Pyramids as that is quite the time to see them, however we got up at 6am & had a guide from the Hotel, went out by train as far as Mena House, & then got camels to ride. Laugh, I laughed till I nearly fell off, on the way back, none of the sisters had ever been on anything before that went without wheels well, we wanted to catch a certain train & had lingered too long round the Sphinx & the pyramids, & had to trot, then the fun began. The Arabs were running along picking up various articles such as hats, kodaks, gloves, bags which were strewn along the road, while the Sisters made violent efforts to hang on, oh but it was too lovely. The Arabs themselves were nearly doubled up, tho they must be used to such sights, & saw such thousands of things I want to take snaps of; have got a good many & do hope they turn out well. Then we got back into Cairo in time to go to the two chief Mosques & the Citadel before lunch. One Mosque we went into they tied on huge slippers before we were allowed to enter, it was a most beautiful place, but did not come up to the Monreale*

Cathedral or the Cappella Palletma in Sicily, the other one is very ancient, & they shewed [sic] *us holes in the wall made by cannon balls fired by Napoleon. I want to get a book on Egypt, then we went back to the hotel & had our lunch, & then once more went forth to the Arab Bazaars, most wonderful places, really filthy & all that, the street just wide enough to walk single file at times, & the wee shops just about three feet by three, with the most wonderful things in them, beautiful brass work & copper things it was no use buying things, had no-where to put them, & it was no use humping them out to Mesopotamia & back … The bazaars were too fascinating for words, but I wouldn't like to wander thro there alone, just like a rabbit warren, for all the world …*

Oceans of love from Narrie

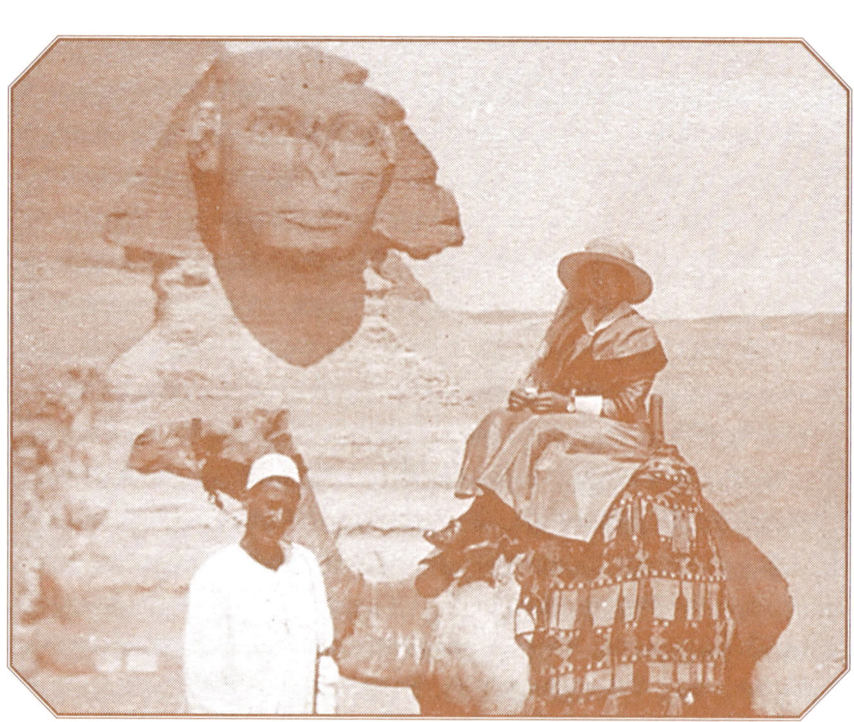

Narrelle on a camel ride at the pyramids, Giza, 1916. (*Hobbes Collection*)

AFTER TEN DAYS OF UNCERTAINTY AND MORE THAN ONE FALSE START, THE 22nd Stationary Hospital was finally on the move. On Friday 28 May, the nurses were woken up at 6am and, after a rushed breakfast, were taken in ambulances to the station for the next instalment of their journey to 'Meso'. As Narrelle explained to her family, the Egyptian hospital train they travelled on was:

> *...a thing of beauty, all dazzling white & red crescents & at 9am we once more started off on our journey 'further East'. The first part of the line lay along the Cairo route, as far as Zantara, I think it was, & then we entered the Mahig Abu Hammad desert, great scot, the heat & dust & sand, it was awful, too awful when we thought of those dear men stationed away out. At Tel-el-Kebir we passed a huge camp, Australians & English, they cheered & waved madly to us as we passed, & I wondered if any of our boys were among them, it was desperately hot & the glare was just awful, they were mostly getting around in shorts & a singlet, helmet & boots. I was frightfully keen to get on to Ismailia for a 4th A.L.H. boy had told me he had just heard that the 6th were at that place, & I had wired to Holt on the offchance of his getting it, & getting to the train, & I was feeling most awfully excited at the thought of perhaps seeing him, & perhaps Tonie, & when the first camps came in sight, I got out on the platform so as not to miss anything, & my dears that rotton Hospital train just sailed through Ismailia camp as tho it simply wasn't there. Australian boys rushed out of every tent, dear shouting, waving, cheering Australian boys, brown as any old Egyptian, I could have just howled, & it was all left behind in a few short minutes. Then my one hope lay in Suez.*

The ambulance train pulled in to Suez at 4.30 in the afternoon. The train station was directly opposite the wharf. Within half an hour, they had boarded their ship, the *Loyalty*, and were sailing down the Gulf of Suez and out into the Red Sea. Narrelle did not meet up with any of her friends in the AIF. She cabled Holt Hardy, Tonie Hordern and others who were still in Egypt, somewhere in the desert, to see if they could arrange a rendezvous. But it was not to be. Either cables were missed or did not arrive in time for the organisation required. Upset, Narrelle attempted to shrug it off.

> *I sought up & down wharf & platform for an Australian uniform. We were dumped out of the train & straight across into the 'Loyalty' & by 5pm we were moving out from the wharf, & I just shed a tear to think I'd been in Egypt nearly two weeks & had not found one man. Out of all the humans I knew there, & there I was starting off for, the lord knows where, it was rotten, & I had planned how I would write Mrs Hardy & tell them how Holt looked etc, & we would yap till our tongues ached, such is life — in the army —*

The *Loyalty*, a hospital ship that ran between Bombay, Suez, the Persian Gulf and Mesopotamia, was originally called the *Empress of India* and belonged to the Canadian Pacific Railway Co. During the war, it was purchased by an Indian maharaja, and renamed *Loyalty*, as a testament to the patriotic loyalty of India towards Britain. Narrelle enjoyed the trip down the Red Sea. She did not get off at Aden as it was extremely hot and they were hovering on the edge of the monsoon, which made the weather humid and unsettled. She had seen enough of Middle Eastern cities. She preferred to keep cool, sitting and reading under a big fan, resting up for the next instalment of her war service — Bombay.

THEY REACHED BOMBAY, NOW CALLED MUMBAI, EARLY ON THE morning of Tuesday, 8 June 1916. The monsoon had broken and it was pouring with rain and extremely humid. Once a series of islands, the city expanded over the centuries into one of India's busiest metropolises, with extremes of wealth and poverty. From 1858, when India came under the full control of the British crown, and through the second half of the nineteenth century, Bombay developed into a major economic centre.

Home for the foreseeable future for Narrelle was the Taj Mahal Hotel, a huge, rather exotic and luxurious hotel on the edge of the harbour. Today the Taj Mahal is still one of Mumbai's finest hotels, a landmark reminiscent of times past, facing the famed Gateway of India, opened in 1924 to commemorate the visit of King George V and Queen Mary. During World War I, the hotel was turned into a convalescent home for officers as well as housing the hundreds of nurses rushed to India to assist with the Mesopotamian campaign.

On arrival in Bombay, Narrelle and her colleagues discovered that the plans to send nurses to Mesopotamia were on hold due to the intense summer heat and adverse weather conditions there. Apart from the small contingent of nurses with the 23rd Stationary Hospital, British nurses were refused permission to go to 'Meso' until the situation improved. But one could hardly recommend Bombay in the monsoon

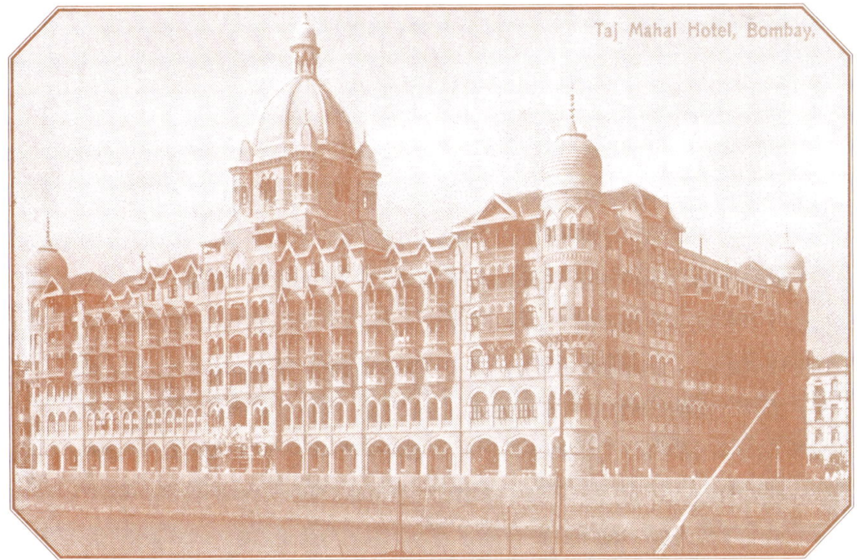

The large Taj Mahal Hotel on the Bombay waterfront became a convalescent hospital and nurses' home during World War I. (*Mary Evans Picture Library*)

either. The best time to visit Bombay is between October and February, when the skies are blue and the weather generally balmy, warm but not oppressive. The monsoon, from mid-June to September is hell on earth, especially if you are not used to it. There is very high humidity with almost no change between night and daytime temperatures of around 80 degrees Fahrenheit (27 degrees Celsius). The average rainfall in July alone is a huge 37 inches (970 millimetres).

During the monsoon, most of the British residents escaped to the hill stations of Simla; Darjeeling; or Matheran, the closest hill station to Bombay; and the entire local government relocated to Poona, over 120 miles (192 kilometres) away, to the south-west of Bombay. Few remained in Bombay and fewer were expected to undertake the physical tasks required by nurses in their day-to-day routine. Small wonder then that Narrelle was hot, bothered and distinctly out of sorts the entire time she was there. Again she railed against the rules and regulations of the British military, and how it treated single female nurses within the essentially male army environment. She hated the English matrons and their 'bally' rules. She described how expensive India was and how they received conflicting instructions about what type of 'kit' to buy for Mesopotamia. Most particularly, Narrelle expressed her hatred of the city during the monsoon. Here was a woman who had spent much of her life in western New South Wales and knew what heat was. Or so she thought. She had also spent last summer in Malta, which had a hot Mediterranean climate. But nothing prepared her for the energy-sapping, debilitating monsoon. It made her feel physically unwell. She tried to describe it in a letter home written from the Taj Mahal Hotel on 10 June.

> *The Monsoon had broken, arrived or any other old thing that a monsoon does, especially rain, 5 inches in 5 hours sort of thing, & I have no hesitation in saying that the monsoon is damned moist and uncomfortable, perspiration did you say? Phew, it fairly pours off you. I've honestly felt the filthiest beast I've ever felt, since I came here, it rolls off you, cheerfully at the slightest movement, & we are all praying to be sent on to*

Mesopotamia. For one thing we will be absolutely bankrupt if they leave us here, another thing up there it's a dry heat, more like our West, & there is work to be done, which is more than one can say for Bombay, however that's another story ... We stayed on board [the *Loyalty*] *till 11am & then we were yanked up here to this wonderful Hotel in ambulances, there seemed to be thousands of Sisters here when we got in ...*

Taj-Mahal is fairly on the edge of the harbour, a huge place. I must get some P.C.'s of it, it's a beautiful building, the floor is rather wonderful, it's composed of broken china, every bit of china is saved & put in with cement, it really looks most quaint, reminds me of a very pebbly beach when a wave has just washed over & left them shiny, & patterns have been made with the different colours, heaven only knows how long it took to do it, as my bedroom is 522 & there are dozens more, besides all the various lounges, dining rooms, halls & everything else, they would be delightful floors out in places where dust storms arrive, for they always look shiny & cool, & just out from our 'duty room' is a heavenly spot, garden, with cocoanut [sic] *trees & palms.*

Alas when we arrived we were informed that for the present the 22nd Stationary was to be left in Bombay. In fact they had taken two floors in the left wing, & were running a Convalescent Home for Officers, & here we are, all bitterly disappointed from our C.C.s down, for there is work to be done in Mesopotamia, heaps of it, & they won't send us up because they say it's too hot 103 degrees & dry if they only knew, it would be infinitely better for us than this, for I don't mind telling you we are fed up with things, it's simply another 'Sicily' which is very sad, & the money we have spent getting things, is too awful, & not all Gov money either which is the worst of it. When we got our orders in Malta we were given £15 to get our campkit & outfit, & told what we were to have in the way of uniforms, which we got. Then when we got to Alexandria & under a different command, we had orders to get all sorts of other things, veils, sou-wester, cooking utensils, spine pads, white shoes & goodness knows what, all of which had to come out of our pockets, oh & food, tinned foods enough to last for three days on arrival in Basra, that also had to come out of our pockets. Then we got here & found we were not to dream of wearing veils, our food stuff is sitting probably rotting in this heat, we are not to wear our overalls while working here, only if we go to Meso — spine pads useless, & a few other fool things, if we go to Basra we have to get another kind of helmet, that's a sample of things, as they are in wartime. Oh & another thing, we had to provide ourselves with turndown collars, & on arrival here were all 'told off' for wearing such bold unladylike, fast things as turndown collars. I tell you we wish to goodness they had left us in Malta. Miss Stow & I have volunteered for Mesopotamia, simply to get away from Bombay & the powers that be, for they have absolutely insulted us, as a unit more than we ever have been before.

I longed to be able to write short hand, to take down the lecture we received the day we arrived. I'd had it all, pretty much the same over in Sicily, but it was all new to the others, & how they hated it, poor girls, mind you not from the Indian side, but from the people who have been sent out from England, for we don't belong to India, I'm sure I don't know what sort of women they take us all for, but, once more, Thank goodness I'm an Australian. But there stop grousing, only, I wish we had an Australian or two at the head of things. I am sitting writing this on duty, there is absolutely nothing to do, it's 6pm & I've not seen my patients since 10am. As soon as the Dr had been round, they went out, & are still out most of them, the rest are, anywhere, there is not a dose of medicine to be given, or a temperature to be taken, out of the whole 43, but we are 'doing our bit' oh yes, & in the years to come, when asked what we did in the great war, can say worked in Malta, wintered in Sicily & Egypt, & 'monsooned' in India … Oceans of love darlings, am awfully well & feel very fit.

Yours lovingly Narrie

Narrelle was not posted to Mesopotamia until late August, so she spent a very frustrating two months languishing in Bombay, through the peak of the monsoon. It was even too hot to write letters. Narrelle found that when she tried to write, her hand stuck to the pen, the paper, and the desk *in a most absolutely disgusting way*. Although Narrelle had experienced harsh conditions in Malta, issues of femininity, appearance and female decency came to the fore in Bombay largely through the oppressiveness of the climate. Additionally most white British women did not 'work' at any time, whereas nurses were working long shifts which demanded high levels of physical exertion, in long dresses made of woollen materials, and layers of clothing — petticoats, bloomers, skirts and the like. The heavy ankle-length dresses and petticoats weighed her down, blouses with starched collars and cuffs cut into her neck and wrists, her feet swelled in her leather shoes, and her stockings were damp with continuous perspiration trickling down her legs.

Narrelle also commented that she and all the nurses were losing their hair and going bald. She believed it was the hard water. This problem was distressing for everyone. Narrelle's hair had gone quite white during her first year of active service. She often mentioned the state of her hair and her quirky remedies in her letters. Her potions included soaking the hair in coconut oil, quinine and castor oil. The problems the nurses had with their hair loss were probably due not only to the climate and work-related stress, but also diet. Because of the monsoon, everything from bread to rice went mouldy very quickly. Narrelle found the food quite unpalatable and described the eggs as tasting of 'earth'. She also found that her stomach did not agree with too much tropical fruit such as paw paws, bananas and especially mangoes, and Narrelle longed for Australian fruit such as apples and oranges. She regularly took an iron tonic supplement to keep up her strength and health, and her general physical constitution was good, despite the odd stomach upset.

> *Darlings you will have to be satisfied with PCs as this heat continues, it's too deadly for words and too hot to even go outside once we are off duty. We leak so much on duty with clothes on that by the time we get off our one desire is to strip and get under a fan on our bed and get sufficient*

energy to go on next day, it really is awful. Brewarrina was good compared to this hothouse climate. Some days the atmosphere is so heavy with moisture that you feel you cannot breathe. Poor Miss Stow is always wet right through to her belt her dress always looks as though she had been out in rain even if she is not working.

... Do you know for 24 hours up to 9am today we have had 5 and a half inches and it's been raining at that rate for the last 6 days and all today, you simply can't imagine what it's like. It doesn't just rain it teems, falls, throws itself down as tho the sky had suddenly burst and keeps on bursting so as we have got into a particularly rotten unit four of us are asking for a transfer 'for Mesopotamia or elsewhere in India', and it's more than likely that we will get it. Besides there is simply nothing doing in our Hospital and the last advice from Mesopotamia is that there are hundreds of men up there waiting to get down to hospitals and plenty for the nurses to do so and really we would much rather be there than in this place living at the largest and most expensive place in Bombay. We would go to Basra first if sent to Mesopotamia or Amara, there we hear they are opening up a big hospital a bit higher up.

Although Narrelle grumbled regularly to her family about her nursing colleagues, she did make some good friends. Jessie Stow — her full name was Isabella Jessie Philipson Stow — was born in 1877 in South Africa, so she was one year older than Narrelle. Jessie came from a military family with all the menfolk serving in the army. At age eighteen, she began her nursing training at St Bartholemew's Hospital in London. Finishing her training just as the Boer War started, she returned to South Africa in 1899 and served with the Natal Volunteer Medical Corps, and at the Intombi Hospital in Ladysmith. For her work during the Siege of Ladysmith, Jessie received the Royal Red Cross medal. Jessie Stow was just the sort of military nurse the QAIMNS needed, so at the outbreak of war in 1914, she enlisted and served in Malta, Egypt, India and Mesopotamia. Narrelle and Jessie first met up in Malta and became good friends. She stayed on in Africa after the war, first as matron of the Dar es Salaam Hospital, and from 1932 to 1952 worked for the Rhodesian Railways Nursing Service. She died in Northern Rhodesia in 1962.

So after a year of active service with the QAIMNS, Narrelle began to moderate her rabid dislike of the British. Becoming good friends with Jessie Stow and others tempered her intolerance and diluted her earlier diatribes against her colleagues. Colonel Thomas Legg, Narrelle's hapless Sicilian climbing companion, also sought her out whilst in transit in Bombay. He was en route to Mesopotamia where they again would meet up. Legg corresponded with her and kept in touch. After all they had worked together in Malta and Sicily and now Meso, so they had much in common and had shared experiences. Whilst Narrelle still had it in for those in authority, there was a general shift in her attitude towards the British from Bombay onwards. For example, when the first group of Australian nurses from Egypt arrived in Bombay, Narrelle did not comment about wishing to join up with them. Rather she was sad because they had postings and she did not.

In 1916, the British asked the Australian government for nurses to assist in the staffing of its hospitals in India. This was to alleviate the shortages left by nurses transferred to Mesopotamia, as well as to serve the increased hospital workload resulting from the campaign. Over 550 Australian nurses, either as part of the AANS or seconded to the British QAIMNS, served in India during the war. Many of them worked in the Victoria War Hospital or at other major medical institutions in Bombay, such as the Colaba War Hospital and the Cumballa War Hospital. Some staffed the hospital ships which sailed from Mesopotamia to Bombay. Others were stationed in hospitals across the Indian subcontinent.

The group Narrelle met arrived in Bombay in July on the hospital ship *Neuralia*. In charge was Matron Emily Hoadley who, like Jessie Stow, had served in the Boer War. These Australian nurses had been working in Egypt and, whilst experienced in military nursing, were worn out from their war service. Two of the nurses contracted cholera and died shortly after arriving in Bombay. Kathleen Power, in her late twenties, was originally from Kilkenny in Ireland. A Catholic, she enlisted with the AANS and embarked from Melbourne with the 10th AGH on 24 August 1915. She died on 13 August 1916 at the Colaba War Hospital. Staff nurse Amy O'Grady was 39 when she enlisted in the AANS. She embarked on the same ship as Kathleen, and died the day before her, on 12 August, just two weeks short of a year since leaving Australia. Amy was survived by her brother, a Catholic priest from Preston, Victoria. Originally both nurses were buried in the Sewri Cemetery, Bombay, but in the 1960s the Commonwealth War Graves Commission relocated all its graves to the Kirkee War Cemetery near Poona.

The remainder of this group was seconded to various hospitals across India, such as Agra, Quetta, Simla and Lucknow. They only lasted about six months in India before being transferred to England. The women were simply unable to withstand the challenging work environment due to the unforgiving Indian climate. Whilst the Australian government allowed its nurses to work in India, it refused to send them on to Mesopotamia as it believed the weather and physical conditions were too extreme for women.

IF THE CIRCUMSTANCES HAD BEEN DIFFERENT AND IF SHE HAD NOT ARRIVED in Bombay in the monsoon, then Narrelle may well have appreciated the city more. For when she did get out and do some sightseeing, she enjoyed what Bombay had to offer. The main sites of interest were the Bombay Zoo, the Victoria Gardens, and the Prince of Wales Museum. Malabar Hill is one of the exclusive parts of Bombay, with wonderful views and slight breezes, where the governor and other dignitaries had palatial houses. Members of the Parsee sect do not bury or cremate their dead as they hold water, earth and fire sacred, so as Narrelle explained:

> [I had] *a delightful motor drive or two round Malabar Hill, where the towers of Silence live, you know the place where the Parsee people bury*

their dead. They are large, round towers open at the top, & inside they have marble tables. The dead are carried up, just wrapped in a white sheet, by two or four 'carriers' also dressed in white, they lay the body on the marble tables, &, uncovering it, close the door. They then go to a hut & take off their white robes, leaving them with the covering from the body, in the grounds where they are, I believe, burnt, for they are never allowed to be taken out of the enclosure having touched a dead body, & new ones have to be supplied for the next funeral. A few hours (three or four) after the body has been deposited on the table, not an ounce of flesh is left on the bones, they have been picked clean by the vultures, & the bones are then removed & burnt. You see the great fat loathsome vultures sitting round the top of the towers.

Malabar Hill itself is most beautiful, & you get a wonderful view of Bombay from the top, you know Bombay is an island, I never realized that before, certainly in one part the distance between the mainland & the town is so narrow that it is spanned by the railway bridge. Then there is another very pretty place, Colaba, a purely garrison point; the old Garrison Hospital is on it, & it has huge old trees very like our Moreton Bay figs. Gov House is at the end of Malabar Hill, but as I before remarked, Bombay is rather beautiful, if only there were not such hordes of natives in every spot. There is not one single place to go to, to get away from them, it's beastly, & how we will enjoy getting back to a place where everyone speaks English, & understands what you want.

When it was not teeming with rain, Narrelle also ventured out into the Bombay streets, and enjoyed the hustle and bustle of an Indian market. She found things very expensive and did not intend to shop but simply enjoyed the whole atmosphere and experience. She also had her friend Jessie Stow to accompany her, which made all the difference.

Miss Stow and I went into the markets one day, a most wonderful place a seething mass of native humanity with most wonderful tropical fruits and vegetables and native flower sellers, stringing poor plucked buds of jasmine and a flower very like the tuber rose on long strings and doing them up into balls and then again fixing them on to a half hoop of silver wire to go round the head. Most quaint, I tried to take some snaps but am afraid there was not enough light and it's always so dull here I can't get any very good ones but I must try one fine day for we ought to be able to get some rather good ones.

Narrelle and twenty other nurses from her unit were temporarily seconded to the Victoria War Hospital. One of the main military hospitals in Bombay, it was located near the docks, and received the most serious cases from the Mesopotamian campaign. The four-storey building had 200 beds on each of the first three floors, with a nurses' quarters on top. Narrelle was allocated to the dysentery ward, which had some of the prisoners exchanged after the fall of Kut. Their condition was heart breaking. She was generally circumspect in discussing her patients, but in Bombay Narrelle let her guard down and was quite graphic.

Oh, the poor emaciated souls, you could learn the bones of the body easily from their frames. I can liken them only unto Indian famine people, or like dead horses on the plains, with the hide just stretched over bones. I'm afraid one is going to die, he is dreadful to look at really, I've never seen such desperately emaciated human beings in my life, & their skin seems so parched & dry, poor dears.

She also began to reminisce about her experiences on Malta and let slip some of her reactions to what she had seen and dealt with during the Gallipoli campaign. Narrelle was greatly affected by her nursing experiences but this was the first time that she attempted to describe her feelings to her family in any detail. She talked about blotting out what she had witnessed to dull her feelings just in case she saw someone she knew. Narrelle referred to the lists printed in the newspapers which detail the fate of soldiers. As a front line nurse, she knew full well what 'wounded' really meant. As she wrote to her family:

The very word 'wounded' is enough to strike horror to the heart of anyone who has seen a shipload of 'wounded' arrive. I'll never forget those first months at Malta, those awful convoys it was the sort of thing that got right on your brain and blotted out everything else and the horror that perhaps the next one you looked at might be one of your own, it seems almost too good to think they might have the same luck Tonie and Holt and some of the others had at Gallipoli.

One way of blotting out these dark thoughts was to focus on her one passion: letters. Both writing and receiving letters from home and from her friends in the AIF was a major source of mental nourishment for Narrelle, and crucial for her psychological wellbeing. Whilst the mail was very erratic and she went weeks without any post at all, when it did arrive, Narrelle was ecstatic. It never got any easier for her. Letters remained her lifeline to the outside world throughout her war service. Even the harrowing monsoon could not dampen her enthusiasm for mail. On 10 July, she wrote:

My darling peoples,

Truly was I overcome with gladness last week when a sister came up from the Taj Mahal Hotel & handed me a bundle of letters, & then again I received two more bundles in the evening, 44 in all, think of it, of course I was on duty all day till 8.30pm & too busy to even open one, & they fairly burnt holes in my table till I could get off, they were perfectly heavenly, & I was the envy of the Hospital. I read myself nearly blind the first night, & then I could not get at them till the next afternoon, when I fortunately had a half day. I retired to my room as soon as I could, turned my fan full on, took off all my clothing, at least with the exception of singlet & tusson bloomers, & lay down on my bed, surrounded by letters. I went at them most methodically & sorted out each group, Home, Jean, Josie–Kit–Grace, Annie, then outsiders letters, then I sorted out the dates & made them come in proper order, after which I sighed & bogged in, & was still bogging in, fairly wallowing in them, at 10pm, letters dated from end of Feb to your latest Els 11th June, & I'll try & answer them by degrees ...

It makes me wonder what it feels like to be cold when you speak of winter, it's so long since I felt it that I've almost forgotten what the sensation is like, the heat here is evil, but nothing to what it is in other places, they tell us there is only a sheet of tissue paper between the trenches in Mesopotamia & the place where they don't make ice.

I hear it is possible that all Australians are now being sent to England to finish their training instead of Egypt, which means France. I'm not sure where I would rather think our boys were, sometimes when I look at these poor souls, emaciated with much dysentery (my two poor Kut men have died & two others) & breaking out in most awful boils, I say to myself, thank heavens our men are not out here, & then I think of some of the ghastly sights, & poor maimed men we had in Malta, & wonder if there is much to choose between for them.

In almost every letter home, Narrelle mentioned Frank Webb. Either she talked about how she had not received a letter from him or she discussed his movements, what he was doing, and how he was feeling. Frank was with Jim Langwell and by this stage, mid-1916, they were in France, a world away, in the middle of the battle of the Somme. Holt Hardy and Tonie Hordern, two other frequent correspondents, remained in Egypt with the ALH.

I had a pet of a letter from poor old Frank last mail. I think reading between the lines that he was feeling very homesick. He had received no Australian letters for months, his last was 4 months old and all the news he had received was gleaned from my letters which by the way all the boys seem to receive, even when they don't get their own home letters. So I always pass on any I get but my last ones were devoid of news as I had not received any myself. Frank said they had been away at a gas school for a few days, they generally send them before they are sent right to the front poor dears. Frank says he now has great confidence in the gas helmets they are issued with for preventative against gas …

I also had quite a long letter from Holt. They are still in Egypt and he begged me to cable to him when we are going back to England for we will have to go either through the Canal or across from Suez to 'Alex' and we won't be in India always and as far as he can see the A.L.H. will be on the Canal till the end of the war which please heaven won't be long, poor dears. Tonie had ridden over to see him a few days before on old 'Doctor' his 'Weil' [Weilmoringle] *horse, both looking very fit. Holt said they had been asked to recommend men to go to England and go through a course of gunnery and qualify for Commissions in the R.F.A. Tonie's name had gone in 'so he has a good chance of having a fair time before he has any more fighting and then as an officer'.*

Tonie Hordern did go on officer training and ended up as a lieutenant. Both he and school friend Alex Guthrie were promoted to lieutenants just before Christmas on 23 December. Narrelle also heard that Ted Nott, another jackaroo from 'Weilmoringle', had been killed in action on 13 July 1916 in France. He had enlisted in the King's Own Yorkshire Light Infantry. A second lieutenant, he was posthumously awarded the Military Cross. Leslie Dill, another young 21 year old from Condobolin who was jackarooing at Brewarrina, had enlisted in June 1915 with the 3rd Infantry Battalion, AIF. He landed on Gallipoli on 7 December, right at the end of the campaign and later served in France. He was wounded on 26 July 1916 with a gunshot wound to the right leg during the battle of the Somme. As Narrelle said, *the boys in Egypt are grousing at being left there but at least they are safe for a time.*

AFTER CELEBRATING HER 38TH BIRTHDAY ON 21 AUGUST, NARRELLE finally received orders to head for Mesopotamia. The arrival of the north winds, or *Shamal*, cooled the place down, and the authorities now deemed it suitable for English nurses. Narrelle was not quite sure where she was going, and to which hospital she was to be posted, but she did not care. To get out of Bombay, and leave the 'moist heat' and incessant heavy rain behind was all she could think of. She was ready for the next instalment of her war service.

Mesopotamia

Chapter 7

'I FEEL LIKE AN EMU SHUT UP IN A 10 BY 10 YARD'

MESOPOTAMIA, NOW IRAQ, IS AN ANCIENT LAND WHICH FOR HUNDREDS of years was part of the large and once dominant Ottoman Empire. The country is largely flat desert fed by two great rivers, the Tigris and Euphrates. Alongside these two rivers are fertile plains and small villages built above river level to help prevent flooding, which inevitably occurs each year as the snows melt in the northern mountains. The two rivers converge at Qurna, 40 miles (64 kilometres) north of Basra, to form the Shatt-el-Arab, a mighty river basin flowing into the Persian Gulf. At the time of World War I the rivers were the lifeline of the region. With few roads, railways or other infrastructure, they became the main form of transportation linking the city of Baghdad, over 500 miles upstream (800 kilometres) on the Tigris River, to the Persian Gulf.

Narrelle's arrival in Mesopotamia was part of the revitalised and reformed medical initiatives for the campaign. From the beginning of 1916, waves of fresh nursing staff, more medical equipment, and mobile hospital units were transported to Mesopotamia, from India, Egypt and England. Thousands of well-resourced and well-trained troops were also brought in to reverse the ignominious defeat of Kut. The whole campaign was transformed. Of course, there were still the long river journeys for the ill and wounded; the climate was still unforgiving with raging heat in summer, heavy rains in winter, and floods, powerful winds and fierce dust storms, mosquitoes, fleas, and flies; but the medical facilities were much improved, the medical treatment was better, and lives were saved. However, it was still incredibly primitive even by contemporary standards. There were none of the modern amenities that we now consider obligatory. Hospitals were bare, miserable places with no airconditioning, only punkas — large fans used extensively in India, and pulled for hours on end by small boys and camp followers to provide some ventilation and breeze.

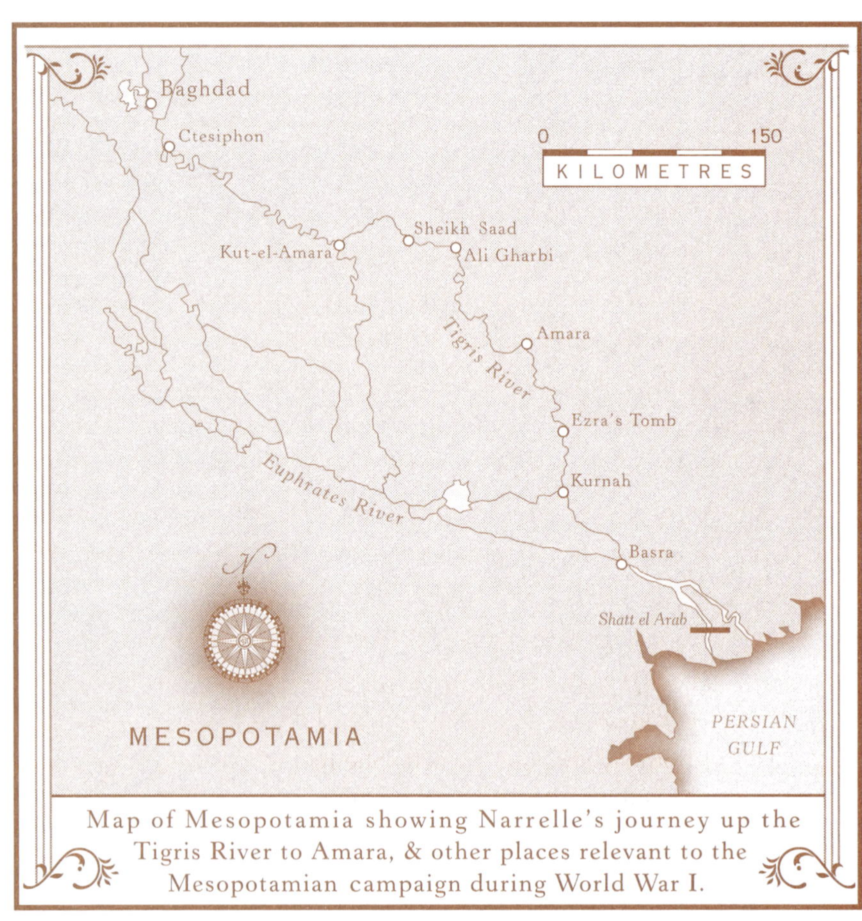

Map of Mesopotamia showing Narrelle's journey up the Tigris River to Amara, & other places relevant to the Mesopotamian campaign during World War I.

NARRELLE WAS REALLY EXCITED ABOUT THIS NEXT 'ADVENTURE'. SHE WAS desperate to leave Bombay and be useful. The war continued to rage with no end in sight and, after fifteen months on active service as a military nurse, Narrelle felt she still had much to offer. A new level of maturity pervaded her extensive and lengthy correspondence from Mesopotamia. There are about 30 letters, many of them very long, descriptive missives. Narrelle spent more time in 'Meso', as she called it, than any other theatre of the war. She arrived in Basra in early September, transferred to Amara in October 1916, and remained there, without any leave, until June the following year, when she was invalided to Bombay.

Through these letters we see a changed Narrelle. She becomes more settled and content within herself, accepting of her situation, although she still lashes out at the British, their unnecessarily strict military rules (as she sees them), and their 'bally' regulations. She never loses her sense of humour though, or her cutting wit. Narrelle had made some good friends, such as Jessie Stow and Thomas Legg, and it was these new wartime friendships which sustained and supported her, and made her war service bearable. She did not write so much about being lonely, a feature of her Sicilian sojourn, but there was still an inner loss, a hankering for the Australian bush, a yearning for the western plains of New South Wales. She was missing a sense of place, a sense of where she belonged. But there was also a growing sense of contentment within herself, as she finally accepted that she would never make it to France and nurse Australian soldiers again, and that it was here, in 'Meso', that she might well stay for the remainder of the war.

Her first letter was written from Basra on 5 September 1916. Despite the fact that it was very, very hot, with temperatures well over 105 degrees Fahrenheit (41 degrees Celsius), Narrelle liked Basra, compared with the soggy, humid Bombay she had just left. She had sailed from Bombay on the *Varsova*, a hospital ship that ran from India to Mesopotamia. One of the earlier complaints in the campaign had been the lack of suitable vessels to transport those invalided from Basra to Bombay. So designated

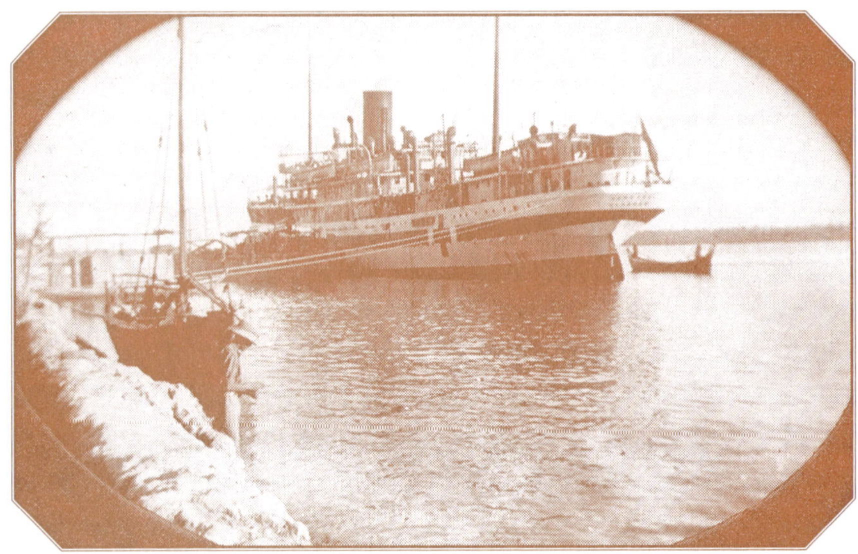

The hospital ship *Varsova* at the mouth of the Tigris River, which ran from India to Mesopotamia. (*Hobbes Collection*)

hospital ships were seconded to the route, staffed with medical teams based in India. Ever since the British troopship *Marquette* was torpedoed off Salonika in the Mediterranean in October 1915 with the loss of ten nurses and nineteen members of the New Zealand Medical Corps, all medical units were transported in hospital ships.

Narrelle was violently sea sick on the five-day voyage through the Arabian Sea and Gulf of Oman, up to the Shatt-el-Arab. She spent three days confined to her cabin, lying in bed feeling decidedly sorry for herself. On arrival in the Shatt-el-Arab, the heat hit Narrelle like an out of control sauna.

> *My beloved peoples never shall I forget the heat of that day and yet it was cool to what they have had it. While we were waiting our turn to enter the river to go up to Basra — and the unknown — a fierce wind arose it was something like those raging days up at Brewarrina with the sky a sort of smoke blue and a wind blowing over the plains of — the place where they don't sell ice — you know when you would crawl indoors,*

shut out every chink of light and pant on the floor with the thermometer standing at 116 or 119 that would give you some little idea what it was like — I wanted to retire to my cabin under a fan but there were so many intensely interesting things to see I jolly well stayed right where I was and took snap shots. Why positively the tar stuff in the cracks on the ship floor was melting and sticking to the sole of your shoe, it's no wonder everyone turns black out here. I'm turning black myself and I can feel the skin on my face positively getting like parchment, oh!

It's some place but I feel quite different up here in this dry heat but this I will say, if it was as hot as this for Adam and Eve in the Garden I don't wonder Eve ate an apple from the tree of Knowledge if she thought she would learn how to keep cool even tho she did only wear a fig leaf. Oh the hot burning glare of it all but I like it far and away more than Bombay, one never really felt well there and you were always sticky. All the way up the river the date trees grow right to the edge of the bank which only seems to be about 3 feet high in most places, not that when the tide is up you would not think there would be such a tremendous rise and fall of the tide so far up, in one place we passed two sunken steamers just part of the funnel and masts standing out of water, and further down the Shatt-Al-Arab, we passed Abadan where the oil pipes are carried to from away up in the oil fields — a great barren looking place with huge tanks and pipes all around but most of all I loved the Date trees laden with dates, groves and groves of them. They have been cultivated for hundreds of years and the whole place is one mass of canals, the dates only grow really as far back as the canals go, they are ripe now and all along the river you would see strange looking huts made of a sort of matting and surrounded by a matting fence. They tell us we would never eat another date especially those packed in boxes if we saw how it is done. I could easily believe it, as it is we get dates boiled or stewed for breakfast, dinner and tea and enjoy them, they say they are fattening.

It took all day to reach Basra. Initially Narrelle was posted to the large No 3 General British Hospital that consisted of the main building known colloquially as 'the Palace'.

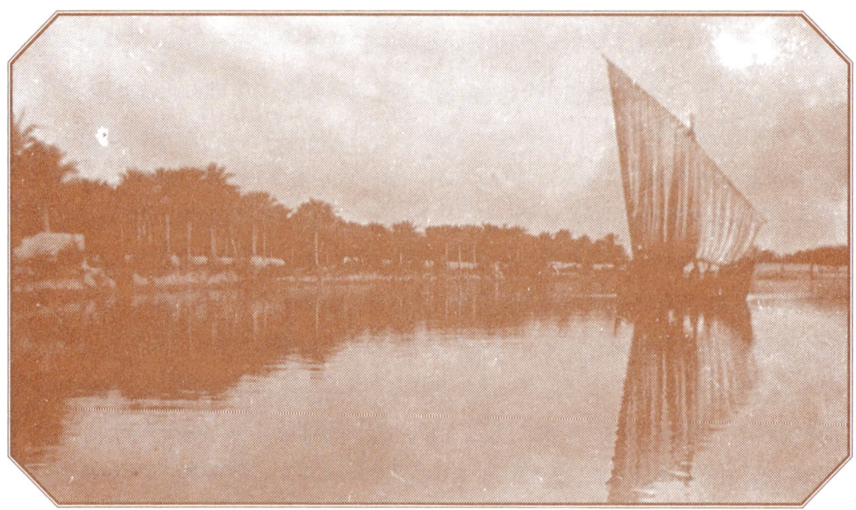

As Narrelle sailed up the Tigris River, she took photographs on her small Kodak camera. Here she captured an Arab sailing ship and date palms reflected in the water. (*Hobbes Collection*)

This was a large and imposing multi-storey structure built on the banks of the Tigris River by the Sheikh of Mohammerah, an Arab leader sympathetic to the British. Around it, nestled on the riverbank, were long rectangular matting huts, with between 24 to 40 beds in each. Narrelle commented on the enteric huts that had electric fans, quite a luxury. There was only a small pathway between the fence surrounding the nurses' quarters and the river. Conditions were still rather primitive and Red Cross supplies were in demand so Narrelle quickly wrote to family friend and Australian Red Cross stalwart Mrs Eleanor MacKinnon for provisions.

Basra, the gateway to Mesopotamia, was a mud-brick town intersected by a series of intricate canals, earning it the nickname, 'the Venice of the East'. The town, originally established by Caliph Omar during his war against the Shah of Persia in AD 637, later became an important trading centre and departure point for Arab sailors and traders dealing with China and India. The hero Sindbad the Sailor, from *The Thousand and One Arabian Nights,* reputedly sailed from Basra.

Predominantly Shi'ite, Basra was the base of early Arab opposition to the Ottoman Empire in the first decade of the twentieth century. The original commercial district was Ashar, which contained the main bazaar and plenty of Arab shops and cafés.

In one letter, dated 4 October, Narrelle described an afternoon trip with a couple of officers into Ashar, where the British had established a Field Force Canteen. The method of transport was generally a *bellum*, a small flat boat pushed by two Arabs with large poles, very similar to a gondola. But the group could not find a *bellum* so the officers suggested walking into Ashar. As Narrelle continued:

> *We had never done so before but having men with us we decided we would, so we ferried over and started off. It was most interesting, we walked away through a date grove past all sorts of strange places and past a native (Arab) village, the building consisting mostly of matting and mud huts and a high matting fence all round it, then on the outskirts of Ashar past a place where Arabs in their quaint robes were winnowing grain, great piles of it ... then on past a cafe where Arabs in dozens were sitting outside on benches and at tables with their Hookah and their coffee absolutely filthy of course. I felt I didn't want to open my mouth to speak because of the filth but it was most quaint they all had their turbans on and different coloured cloaks sort of jibbah shape then we got to the bazaar and went right through.*
>
> *It was really most fascinating, all the wonderful grains and fruits and brilliant hued materials and all sorts of most wonderful things pottery brass ware but oh all so dirty — eugh — and yet it's wonderful how little disease there is amongst them or else we don't hear of it. We passed right through the bazaar from one end to the other and then out along the banks of Ashar creek where they have more and more coffee and soft drink places for Arabs where they sit in hundreds smoking and drinking their various liquids and gossiping.*
>
> *It was too dark to be able to take any snap shots by this time the sun was just down and we had to hurry on, for once the sun goes down it gets*

dark, there is no twilight and we do not like being out after dark, it's safe enough early in the evening but I wouldn't trust an Arab any further than I could see him most times. We wandered around and found the places we wanted then got a bellum and drifted out into the river it was a most perfect evening. Really this is a most fascinating place the glorious colour in the sky shading to a deep purple with intensely bright stars and the feathery date trees against the sky line and quaint most quaint large old bellums that drift down the river and out, carry dates, cases and cases of dates and other things to different ports and even to Bombay.

Until Narrelle acclimatised to Mesopotamia, the heat continued to be the main topic of conversation. The general living and working conditions all round were challenging, to say the least. But she described all in an observant and humorous way.

Forgive pencil, can't help it, ink dried up mostly, like everything else in this land of sun & heat — heat & sun, tho thank goodness it's starting to get cooler now, & the nights are positively cold, which makes it much better, but oh ye gods, the heat has been almost beyond words — I can only liken it unto the white heat of Bourke in mid summer, when you could not get away from it, or into any shade, your eyeballs were parched & tender, & when the wind blew, the dust was as the dust of the grassless plain, oh yes, it's some place, & the women who have been here all through the summer are just wonderful, & the poor men, how I pity them out in the full blast of it, however it will soon be over for a few months & we will be in for all the rain we could wish for.

This is active service for a sure thing this trip, & shall I tell you what I am longing for, a room to myself, clean rain water to wash in, in a real bath — tea with milk, real milk & bread without weavils, butter that is not margarine and real rain water to drink, not stuff that has been doctored up to make it fit for drinking. I told you I could eat tinned things like any old sailor, Biltong like any Boer, Macaroni like a Sicilian, goat & cheese like a Maltese, Buffalo like an Egyptian & Date like an Arab, Curry & Rice like an Indian & any other old thing oh it's a great life, & there are a few people who sit around in luxury & have everything to their hand & then grizzle, lord they want a little active (with a capital A) service.

... This is a most quaint place, & yet it somehow reminds me of Brewarrina, it's certainly just the same heat, dry & hot, sort of frizzles up one's outside & the backs of one's eyeballs ... Today my dears is a typical red hot 'back-o-sunset' day, red hot, red hot wind with clouds & clouds of dust, we are breathing it, eating it, thinking it, & our eyes are blinded by it, while across the river, at the back of the fringe of date trees, you can see clouds & clouds of pale yellow dust rising up from the desert, beyond, you can clean your shoes every time you step outside the doorway, but they are always dirty, & you are always thirsty, oh it's some country.

Oh, this is a quaint place, you go everywhere in a bellum, by water. There are little creeks running everywhere & you are punted up & down. You look at the water in the river & realize that everything gets dumped into it & from that same water we drink — after it has been well chlorinated.

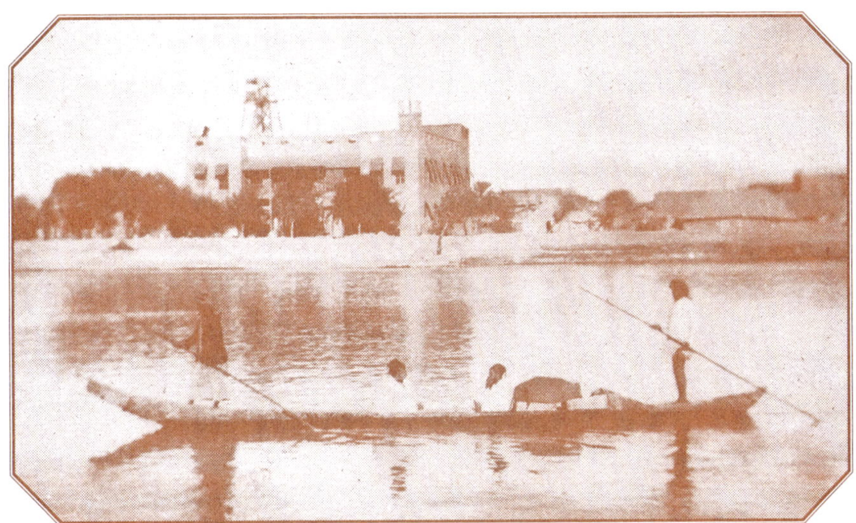

A convalescent hospital with wireless station on top and, in the foreground, a common form of water transport on the Tigris, a *bellum*. (*Hobbes Collection*)

Narrelle continued to focus on receiving, or not receiving as the case may be, her beloved cache of letters. It was the bane of her life not to receive her letters that brought news from a world far removed from war, sickness and the military, a world of family and friends, and familiar places called home. Later on, Narrelle did relax somewhat and finally accepted the peripatetic nature of the mail deliveries. They really were at the end of the world. In Mesopotamia, Narrelle was totally isolated and cut off from not only her world but also from the war. The campaign here was a backwater, far removed from the 'main game' of the western front. People back home in Australia did send her newspapers and magazines such as the *Bulletin* and the *Brewarrina Times*. However, such was the delay with newspapers, Narrelle, for example, heard only from friends' letters about the tragedy of the 1916 Somme battles, especially those involving Australian troops at Fromelles and Pozières. Her frustration at the lack of information was clearly evident. Her isolation was complete.

> *Miss Birt* [in charge of the Red Cross Hospital at Huntington] *told me that some of our Australian regiments have been almost wiped out, poor dear boys, Jean it's just heartbreaking, to think of it, how they must have suffered. I've not had letters from anyone for weeks, Holt or Frank or any of the men who write most regularly, since the Malta days, & we get little or no news here, it's awful. You get up & have breakfast, come on duty all day, or most of day, go off & go to your room, & to bed, & get up the following day & do the same, & so on. We can't go outside the Hospital unless there are two of us, not even out for a row on the river & we may not go into Basra without a man, so, I feel like an Emu shut up in a ten by ten yard.*

She heard from Frank in a letter dated 12 August that he was involved with the Australian artillery in France but was safe. Not so lucky was their friend Geoff Yeomans, who was killed in action. Geoff had been promoted to lieutenant in early March 1916 and was with the 1st Battalion, AIF. He died during the night of 22 July with Major

Lindeman prior to the attack on Pozières. Geoff's body was never found. Narrelle was really distressed. As she wrote home: *I'm awfully sorry to hear of poor Geoff Yeomans death. You know the last year he was in Brewarrina, he completely turned over a new leaf.* She now had three friends who had died in the war: Geoff; Wilfred Hartridge, killed in action at Gallipoli in 1915; and 'little' Ted Nott. It got to the point where Narrelle dreaded looking at the casualty lists printed in the newspapers, even if they were months old, for fear of seeing names of men she knew. She noticed that her young eighteen-year-old half-cousin Reg Hobbs had been wounded, and she related Frank Webb's narrow escape in France.

> *Had quite a long letter from Frank yesterday, dated early in September. They had evidently moved back from the Somme, for he said they had moved from —— at last, and what recollections he had of the place he wished to forget, that it was there Ted* [Nott] *got killed and hundreds of other Australians, and the country around was just covered with graves and unburied bodies, poor souls, it must be ghastly sticking there in front of it all, with the knowledge that there is every possibility of your body remaining there, pretty gruesome, and I think it's wonderful the way they get used to it. Frank said he had had one very narrow shave. He was sitting writing … in the doorway of the gun pit, a puff of wind blew the paper away, and while recovering it three shrapnel bullets hit the place where he had been sitting. If they had been half a minute sooner, he would have stopped the lot, long may his luck stick to him.*

BECAUSE THE WAR WAS PROCEEDING BADLY FOR THE BRITISH, THE authorities tightened up on the censorship of correspondence. On arriving in Mesopotamia, Narrelle noticed a marked change regarding censorship of material and the content of her letters. She discussed this topic quite regularly as she moaned to her family about what she could and could not say in her letters. Due to the disastrous nature of the earlier campaign, British authorities were particularly sensitive to events in Mesopotamia. As Narrelle wrote:

> *My poor old diary is getting filled up but alas I cannot pass on any private opinions, strictly forbidden by censor. We've a list, about a yard long, of things we may not say in our letters, & by the time you have sorted out the things you may not say, it leaves you mightily little you may say, hence my deadly stodgy letters, great saving in note paper but you will have to be satisfied with 'Ramblings of a blind mute'. Those 'service cards' the Australian boys had would meet the case exactly, thus — I am well — I have not (or have) received your letters, I am busy — no that gives too much of the show away, therefore we say I am enjoying — what — but I must admit, joking apart, that I prefer the climate up here to Bombay.*

In her correspondence, Narrelle often commented on current political events in Australia. Perhaps if she could not discuss what she was doing in Mesopotamia, she could have her say on events back home. What her comments reveal are the politics of a conservative woman who had a temper and was intolerant of those who opposed the war. She reflected the position of those in Australia, especially many from the middle classes who vigorously supported the war, and was scathing against those who did not. The home front in Australia during World War I was a place of discord and violence. There was significant strike action throughout the war culminating in the Great Strike of 1917. But as Narrelle responded in a letter, there were many less well-known and well-remembered strikes. For example, in August 1916, a peak time for shearing just before spring lambing, about 2000 shearers in New South Wales went on strike for better wages. Their union, the Australian Workers' Union (AWU), and the Labor Council of New South Wales did not back the strikers, so they turned to the International Workers of the World (IWW), or 'wobblies' as they were known, for support. As Narrelle stated in no uncertain terms:

> *I am so glad to hear you have had so much rain all round — but these rotters of shearers — I have just been reading about them in the British Australian [Australasian] they are the limit without doubt, brutes. I'd like to put every man jack of them yanked off into the firing line it's just the sort of thing that would do them good, & we would get rid of the riff-raff. It just makes my blood boil when I think what men are going through over here, Egypt, France and the others, & those brutes going on like that, gee they want shooting.*

The other major controversy in Australia was the issue of conscription. By mid-1916, the only country involved in the war that had not introduced conscription was Australia. The Australian Labor Party (ALP) had a policy of no conscription. However, after an extensive tour of the western front and England in 1916, Australia's new ALP prime minister, Billy Hughes, decided that in order for Australia to keep up its troop numbers, and most importantly remain as an independent force (and not be mixed in with British regiments), conscription must be introduced. The voluntary recruitment numbers were simply too low to sustain the ongoing carnage of the war. Rather than run the risk of a very public brawl within his party, which would certainly not support conscription, Hughes decided on a plebiscite. He would let the people of Australia decide the issue. After a furious campaign in which the federal government unleashed its full powers of persuasion on the Australian people, the referendum was held in October 1916. To the shock of Billy Hughes and others, it was narrowly defeated. Narrelle conveyed her feelings about the result.

> *We are all very distressed about conscription and all its doings, it's too dreadful. Why in heavens name could not Hughes be a man for once. He had it in his power to simply put his foot down, and say 'yes' it's all those boys, left on Gallipoli, all our regiments that will gradually be wiped out in France till they simply don't exist, simply for the want of reinforcements and the knowledge that there are the men over there to come if*

they only would, that hurts. I wish to heavens a few German ships would get busy over there and blow half Sydney — Melbourne and the other places into ruins, as they have blown places over here, and it might blow a little human feeling into the brutes.

Australia was quite unique during World War I for it had an elected federal labour government at the helm. The Australian Labor Party, formed in 1891, had within a reasonably short space of time become one of the leading political parties. At the outbreak of war, Labor was in power in New South Wales, Tasmania and Western Australia, and from September 1914 at a federal level. The Labor government of Andrew Fisher, then Billy Hughes, also had a huge majority in the Senate. Yet the strain of governing in wartime, and the conscription debate of 1916, led to a split in the party. Hughes was expelled from the ALP and he, and some of his key ministers, negotiated a merger with the opposition party to form the Nationalist Party in January 1917. Billy Hughes retained the job of prime minister, and in May 1917 won a landslide election. As always, Narrelle had her opinion but perhaps she did not realise Hughes' continued role as prime minister.

Oh, my dears, I'm simply overjoyed to hear the result of the Election, to think that the bally labour people are at last out of it, it will be the saving of Australia. Thank goodness people have come, a bit, to their senses. What I do want to see tho is conscription and let them send more and more troops. Of course we are awfully keen to know what Russia intends doing, if she is low-down enough to make a separate peace. Well most of us will find ourselves in Constantinople — or India and all our work will go for nothing, for they will simply swoop down like vultures and — but there it simply must not happen. Good lord, people out there simply don't grasp what it would mean, if all those thousands and hundreds of thousands of soldiers were suddenly let loose from Russia. Our men have been splendid and all that up here, but, they can't do the impossible. But there, only I do, do wish the people of Australia would realize just what it would mean, not only to us, but to them, and to India if we were forced to give up here. Why, apart from the open gateway to the ocean — and they would soon get their submarines across — there are the oilfields at Abadan, and then India, India the home of unrest, India, ready to rise any old time, with her millions of uneducated fanatics. I wish I could just sit down and talk, there is so much to talk about that must not be written about.

IN THE LAST WEEK OF SEPTEMBER, NARRELLE'S GOOD FRIEND JESSIE Stow arrived from Bombay. Much to Narrelle's delight, they would both be transferred upstream together to Amara. Jessie arrived with a very strange story that was circulating in Bombay. There were rumours that Narrelle had been so ill on the voyage over to Basra that she had died and been buried at sea. Narrelle laughed it off and joked that the authorities could not *get rid of me so quickly just yet*. But the story underlined the nature of active service, that there were dangers for nurses, be it in travelling through minefields or submarine-patrolled waters, or succumbing to fatigue and disease in the miserable climate.

The conditions in which Narrelle and her colleagues from the QAIMNS and RAMC worked in Mesopotamia were extreme. The temperatures were often above 115 degrees Fahrenheit (46 degrees Celsius) in summer, and deathly cold in winter and at night, with raging winds, flooding rivers, and rain that instantly turned the place into a muddy quagmire. Insects such as mosquitoes, sandflies, fleas and flies, as well as rats and other vermin all led to immense sickness in the troops. Death through diseases such as dysentery, enteric fever and even cholera was frequent. Other minor illnesses included diarrhoea, jaundice, sandfly fever, malaria, septic sores and sunstroke. Scurvy was particularly prevalent in Indian troops and all cases had to be evacuated to Bombay.

Whilst malaria was the most common reason for admission to hospital for both British and Indian troops, it was the sheer numbers of patients with dysentery and enteric fever that overwhelmed medical staff. Narrelle was used to nursing dysentery and enteric fever; she had seen and dealt with both diseases in Malta and Bombay, and was, by this stage, a very experienced nurse. But it was the scale of diseased patients in Mesopotamia that was most confronting. Dysentery, usually spread by flies (from which you could not escape), inflames the colon. The symptoms are severe diarrhoea and pain. What was termed enteric fever was in fact either typhoid or paratyphoid. Paratyphoid is similar to typhoid with milder symptoms. Typhoid, however, is highly infectious and is caused by ingestion of contaminated water or food. All medical staff were inoculated against typhoid but that still did not prevent infection. Perhaps the most dangerous disease, however, was cholera. A highly infectious epidemic disease, with symptoms of diarrhoea and vomiting, patients could rapidly go downhill, leading to the collapse of the kidneys and certain death.

Although a hardened military nurse by this time, Narrelle was still affected by the deaths of her patients. She described one patient from her ward in Basra who had been recovering well from enteric fever and was slated to go up to Bombay on the next hospital ship and then home to England, as he had been in the army for 25 years. But as she explained, *when I went on duty in the morning I found that during the night he had suddenly developed cholera and had been taken away to the cholera hut, I went straight away to see him, but he was quite unconscious then, it was <u>too</u> sad, and I could do nothing, and he had written his wife telling her he was going to Bombay.*

On Thursday, 5 October, after a month at Basra, Narrelle, Jessie Stow and about eighteen other nurses including their matron-in-chief, Miss Beatrice Isabel Jones, were transferred to Amara, about 130 miles (208 kilometres) further up the Tigris River. From Cheshire in northern England, Beatrice Jones originally trained at St Bartholomew's Hospital, London, and served in the Boer War. Awarded a CBE and RRC for her services to military nursing, she was appointed matron-in-chief for Mesopotamia from 1916. The popular and hard-working matron died in

January 1921 in Baghdad, at the age of 54. She was buried in the Baghdad (North Gate) War Cemetery, which is just outside the north gate of Baghdad city on the road to Baguba.

Their mode of transport up the Tigris River to Amara was a small flat-bottomed boat called the *Malmer*, generally used for bringing the wounded and sick down from the front. The women shared the boat with about twenty officers and an assorted group of Chinese, Indian and Tommy soldiers and labourers. The Indian army was a polyglot of people, cultures, and religions, with Christian, Muslim, Hindu and Sikh. The women were screened off from the men and given a small area on the deck for their baggage and camp beds. They set off at dusk and, as Narrelle wrote:

> *It was simply glorious slipping along up the river, just after the sunset, with a most glorious after-glow and the date trees, feathery against the exquisite orange sky, the colour darkening till it was a most wonderful purple with the stars glimmering like diamonds and the lights of the ships in the Stream and the lights of the hospitals and of Magill, a little village higher up the river, twinkling out.*

They berthed for the night just after midnight near Qurna where the Tigris and Euphrates Rivers meet.

> *The next morning I was awake at dawn and lay watching the daylight come and the sunrise, shining through the stems of the date trees the low grey banks and the most wonderful reflections in the river. Oh it was perfectly gorgeous, the water slipping past us flowing down, the reflections of the palm trees and quaint boats as they floated down stream and then on our other hand Qurna, with its mud walls, palm trees, Arabs in their strange garb, dirty, filthy dirty, women coming to the edge of the river to fill their wonderful water pots and then balancing them sideways on their heads. Most of them with black cloths draped around them for frocks and forming veil and headcovering, they came to the river side to wack their dirty rags and their brass pots and trays, things I yearned to buy …*

... The country along the river is <u>most</u> interesting, here and there you would see an old longhaired, brown and yellow sheep or perhaps it would be a mob of quiet eyed cattle and then you would come to fields and fields of corn and maize, some of it just yellowing. It's a most <u>wonderful</u> grain country, most wonderful, every here and there in the crops you would see weird old men standing on round mud hillocks, like flat topped ant beds. I asked what they were doing and was told they were acting as scarecrows, they certainly looked the part to perfection. At lunch time away in the distance we saw, on the bank of the river a little oasis, palm trees around a few mud walls, and rising from the centre a dome and were told it was Ezra's Tomb and that we would pass right by it so, we got our Kodaks ready. It took us ages to get up to it for the river winds and winds in a truly wonderful way. You would be going along past a cornfield, which apparently stretched for miles and miles but away in the middle of it you would see a large bellum with gleaming sails, calmly sailing over the top and through the grain, while away in another direction altogether you would see a paddle boat apparently sailing over another field, it was quite the quaintest thing possible, and we could pick out our route by the sailing boats over the fields and at one moment you would see an object just over your right side and on looking up from your book or sewing you would find the same object well over your left side so it was with Ezra's Tomb. We seemed to follow it all round the country till at last we got to it, such a wonderful place, there was a sort of small mound of rising ground, with high mud walls enclosing it and on the top of the mound the domed Tomb of Ezra, in the most wonderful shade of blue Mosaic and here and there tall old date palms and by these same waters the exiled captives from the Jewish hill-country across the desert to the west 'sat down and wept'.

Narrelle was mesmerised by her journey up the Tigris River. Never in her wildest dreams did she imagine that she would be undertaking such a trip, to places of such importance to all mankind — to Christians, Jews, and Muslims alike. As they crept past Qurna, she could see the reputed site of the Garden of Eden and, a few miles to the west, the remains of

Babylon and the Tower of Babel. She was in an ancient land and she could feel its power and magic. Immediately she wanted to buy a book on Mesopotamia to read more about the country, to inform and immerse herself in the culture.

Narrelle began reading the *Rubaiyat of Omar Khayyam*, first translated into English in the 1850s. A Persian astronomer, mathematician, philosopher and poet from the eleventh century, Omar Khayyam has been called the poet of destiny. His views on life in terms of one's ability to control destiny and fate influenced Narrelle. Khayyam urged one to go from the external to the internal; to live every moment, not the past or the future. His ideas of not being in control of our life and death resonated with Narrelle, and gave her some inner peace. For there is little doubt that Narrelle did find a certain spiritual equilibrium in Mesopotamia. Through the readings of philosophers like Omar Khayyam, she began to accept her situation more willingly and do the job at hand rather than always wanting to be somewhere else, with someone else. As she wrote:

> *After many days in the East, and much time to myself I am starting to read my Omar over again and find him a delightful companion. I can see him sitting on a bench, or out under the date trees, a cup of grape juice beside him — or his hookah — dreaming dreams in the exquisite sunshine with the blue Persian sky above him, this place fairly fascinates me sometimes, it gets hold of me. Later and the sad part of it is that I will not have anyone to sort of talk things over with and to remind each other of things that happened and compare notes, for you know how nice it is to do that.*
>
> *The evenings here are rather wonderful and always appeal to me. Just now I went out to the Chatthi for some water, and there was the most wonderfully bright, tiny rim of a new Moon, hanging above a most gorgeous orange sky, with the quaint matting huts and the palm trees outlined against it, in the soft purple light and the little silver shape hanging there in a soft opal sky (creamy pink) above the orange and yet*

looking almost transparent just on the other side of the huts, the church bell, an old shellcase softly clanging out, its message for 7pm service, later on, at 9pm it will be dark, so dark that you can almost feel it, with the stars shining like so many million diamonds in a deep violet sky and the Last Post will be sounded by a bugler, each note clear as the note of a bird and the last three notes, rising up, up clear and sustained. I don't know why, but to me those last notes always seem like the Benediction, and instinctively one bows one's head as the last note hangs in the still clear air, clear and flute like.

On and on they sailed, up the Tigris towards Amara. Narrelle sat back on her deck chair and absorbed the scenes slowly passing her. Later she tried to re-create the landscape and its people for her family.

Every here and there we would pass strange native villages, some just like the native villages on the way to Cairo, made of mud with high mud walls with loop-holes in them, all round the village, others consisted of just matting huts, the roof made in the form of an Arab and on each side of the door-way — when there was a door, it was mostly left open and then they were fastened to each side — were fastened bunches of bamboo, or rather palm leaves. The people used to chase along the banks wanting to sell live fowls, eggs and fish that, judging by the stiffness of their anatomy had been dead many days and humped along to the side of many 'P' boats in the sun, till they were fairly baked. The women mostly had nose rings studded with blue stones or beads, and long strings of various coloured beads, the size of marbles, dangling from just above their ears.

Then in one place we were followed by a yelling crowd of Arabs, most of them absolutely in their birthday suits, from infants of 10 years to men of 50. The women mostly had black, brown or a most vivid scarlet cloth wound round them forming dress and head covering, they were absolutely like a lot of animals, yelling out what sounded like 'Camera', 'Camera' and 'Bebe'. 'Bebe' meaning woman, and the inevitable cry of 'Bachshee, Bebe, Bachshee', they ran along the bank of the river for miles, diving into the river and throwing filthy rags on to the boat for you to tie something into, awful brutes ...

In one place we came across a well, being turned by a horse, the shaft thing turning a wheel which in turn, drew up water in sockets round each spoke, (sound most elaborate, eh what) then we came across another, most primitive, a bullock was made to walk up a mound of earth, a rope then fastened round its neck and it was made to run down the mound, at the same time drawing up a pig skin or goat skin more likely, made with a long spout of the skin, out of which the water poured into a trough, as it got to the top.

The Tigris got narrower and shallower the further up they sailed. Punted may be a better word. Between Ezra's Tomb and Qala Salih, appropriately called 'The Narrows', boats could not pass each other, especially during sandstorms, fog or at night. They had to stop and allow the procession of wounded through, which had priority on the waterways. The wind picked up and the boat swayed from one side of the muddy river to the other trying to keep in the deeper channel. At one point the boat was stuck on a mud bank, so two Indians had to get

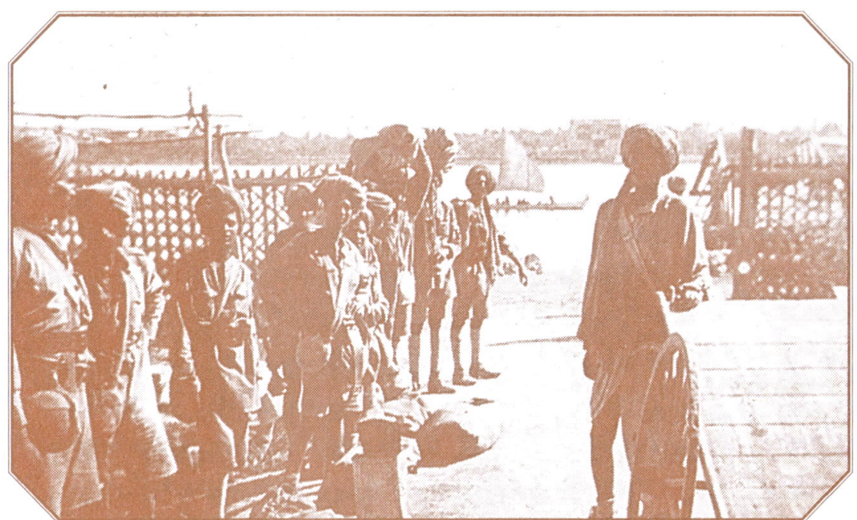

Indian troops, Amara, 1917. (*Hobbes Collection*)

onto the bank and push against it with their feet and backs to dislodge it from the gooey, sticky sludge. They saw gangs of Arabs working on the Basra to Baghdad railway and they passed a couple of convoys heading downstream.

This was one of the visible signs of the improved medical situation in Mesopotamia. It was not until February 1916 that the first hospital ship, the *Sikkim,* arrived in the region staffed by members of the No 20 Casualty Clearing Station. The River Sick Convoy Unit was also formed and given better boats and paddle steamers, improved in design, capability and comfort. The numbers of sick patients sent downstream to Basra from the front for the six months from June to November 1916 included 927 British officers, 12,747 British troops, and almost 25,000 Indians and followers.

On arrival in Amara, Narrelle was allocated to the 32nd British General Hospital, a large sprawling hut and tent hospital on the banks of the Tigris. This was to be her home for the next nine months.

Chapter 8

'THE LAND OF HEAT, FLIES AND DESERT'

THE 32ND BRITISH GENERAL HOSPITAL WAS ONE OF THE MAIN HOSPITALS in Amara. It consisted of huts made from mud and matting, roughly built. Three-quarters of the walls were mud based with reed matting shutters that lifted in and out, abutting the roofs. The roofs were made of a mixture of mud and straw. There was no glass so muslin was used to cover windows. The floors were made of mud hardened by water or cresol. There was no electric lighting in Amara until early 1917 so oil and kerosene lamps were the order of the day. Each hut was divided into two wards holding 88 beds in total, with a small duty room in between each ward. For each hut, there was generally one sister and three staff nurses on duty. A number of male orderlies were also attached to the huts, as well as local Arab boys who were hired to pull the punkas, large canvas structures used to provide a cool breeze for the patients.

Narrelle liked Amara, at this time of year at any rate. The dry heat of October agreed with her. The climate reminded her of Brewarrina, fairly hot in the day, with clear ice-blue skies, and 'glorious' cold nights. Even the dust, which was everywhere, was somehow bearable. It was a soft, grey, light powdery dust into which feet sank up to the ankles. It was a dust which covered everything and everyone, even when the wind was not blowing. It settled lightly, permeating the skin, giving one that never quite clean, slightly gritty, feeling. Tall green date palm groves surrounded the hospital, hugging the river as if their life depended on it. The groves stretched back about one mile, watered by small irrigation channels. Away to the north-east, on the horizon, were the Persian hills, with their snow-capped peaks providing a distinct contrast to the yellow sand and green palm fronds of Amara.

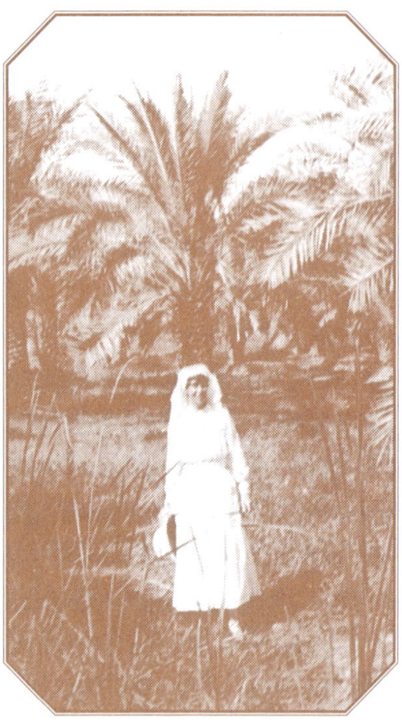

Narrelle among the date palms, Amara, 1917. (*Hazelton Collection*)

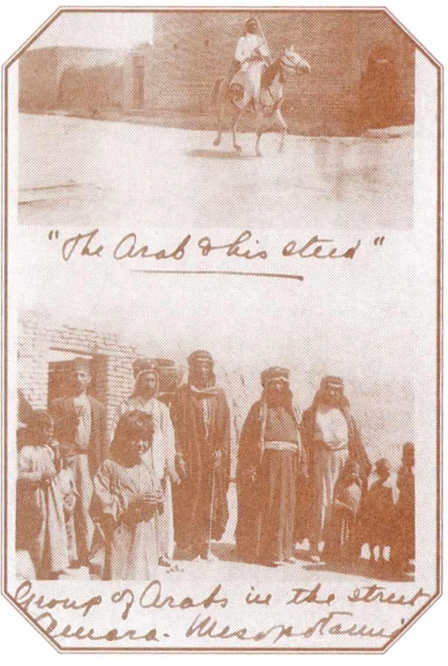
"The Arab & his steed"
Group of Arabs in the street

Narrelle often wrote home describing the local people of Amara. Here her photograph and captions have been made into a postcard, 1917. (*Haskins Collection*)

The 32nd was about ten minutes walk from Amara township, which was spread along both sides of the river, linked together by a bridge of boats that opened at various times. For the nurses to get to the town from the hospital a covered bullock cart called a 'tonga' could be used and there was also a regular launch. But Narrelle generally loved to walk to Amara along the riverbank, with either one or two companions. Nurses were not allowed out of the hospital compound unless in pairs, and if accompanied by a man, then a chaperone was required. Narrelle

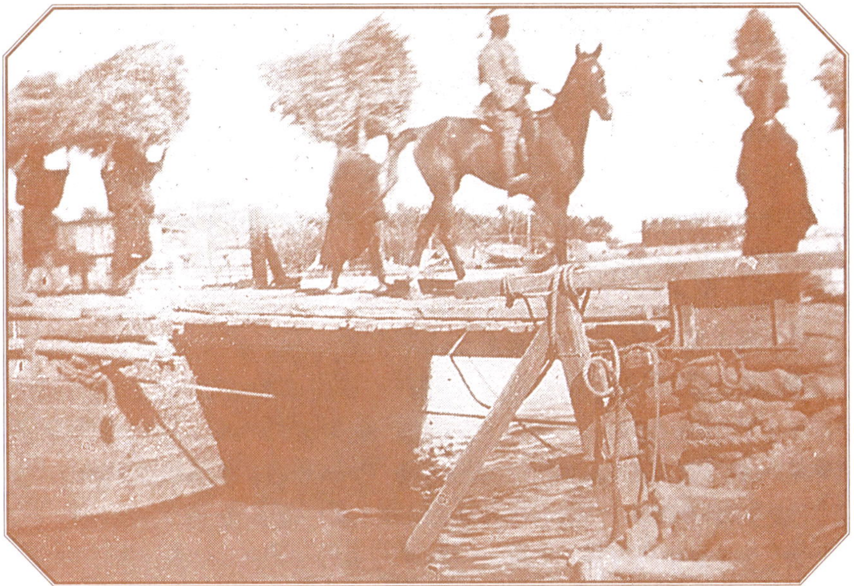

A bridge of boats across the Tigris River, 1917. (*Hobbes Collection*)

particularly liked to walk down around 5.30 in the evening just on dusk. As the sun set over a clump of date tree palms it threw out exquisite reflections and light of varying shades. She also became familiar with the regular Muslim prayer call.

> *It's so weird in the evenings, just at dusk, and in the early dawn, to hear the 'Call of the Faithful', the Muzzien* [sic] *calling from the domes of the various Mosques dotted all round. I could not think what it was for a long time, till someone told me. They just call on two notes, and then it is taken up from Mosque to Mosque and so passed on and then later on, you hear the howl of the jackals, they make a most fiendish noise and come right into the Hospital ground sometimes, they rather remind me of native dogs, only they go about in packs.*

She became an observer of her surroundings and the local people. Narrelle was often very critical of the Arabs, especially their hygiene and living habits, and was both intrigued and appalled at their customs.

Many of her reactions reveal Narrelle to be a product of her time, a white woman of empire, largely ignorant of different cultures and customs, and racist.

> *I must really try and pick up the Arab chant when they are going to their work, it's the quaintest thing possible, and they have something in their hands that makes a noise, like castanets, and you will see a dozen or so little children, from about 4 years up to 13, getting along with their baskets of mud on their heads, singing in quaint rather harsh voices, clacking their hands and suddenly breaking into a sort of dance. Can you imagine wee things like Rona, carrying about eight to ten lbs of mud in a flat kind of basket on their heads to pass up onto the roof of a hut they are building, or re-mudding, and fighting like little wild cats for a basket as soon as it is thrown down empty from the roof and always the colouring is so wonderful; and the women carry themselves so awfully well, they nearly always wear some dark material (if it's not dark originally, it's filthy with dirt) in rags wound or draped around themselves for a dress, but underneath, and showing, at every turn they invariably have some brilliant colouring, red, orange, scarlet for choice, and their dark skins, some of them are really rather fine looking. Nearly every woman has a nose ring of gold studded with turquoise, the turquoise is supposed to be a very lucky stone, and nearly everyone has one somewhere about their anatomy, and you will see tiny children of 7 or 8, with quite fine turquoise nose rings. In India, if a woman displeases her husband, it's quite a common thing for him to bite the end of her nose off with the ring in it. Some of the Indian sisters told me they were continually getting women in hospital with half a nose, and once more I say thank heavens I was born British.*

THE DAY BEGAN WITH *REVEILLE* AT 5.30AM. NARRELLE GENERALLY awoke then (or even earlier at 4.30am as summer approached) and attended to her letters because it was the coolest, and quietest, part of the day. Nurses worked a full shift until 8.15pm with about three hours at most during the day free to do their various chores such as mending, washing, resting, tidying, boot cleaning, the odd trip into Amara, and of course, most importantly, letter writing. During the heat of the day, nursing staff rested, with much activity carried out after sundown.

There was little to do when off duty, apart from eat, sleep, write letters and wander around Amara. Tennis courts and hockey pitches were set up but it was often too hot to play. The food was also limited. Rations consisted of bully beef, bacon, rice, army biscuits, bread, butter, and cheese. Tinned food such as sardines was a staple. They could buy biscuits, fresh fruit — especially dates, chutneys and other condiments — from the canteens and the Amara markets. The main produce of Mesopotamia was wheat, barley, wool, rice and dates so these foods were readily available. Once Narrelle bought a small cake made by the Australian biscuit company Swallow and Ariel at the canteen. It was a tiny sixpenny cake, very expensive, but she longed for cakes and they were such a treat. The British Red Cross opened a depot in Amara which supplied cigarettes, tobacco and other provisions or luxuries not obtainable elsewhere. These were distributed regularly to patients. Australian Red Cross blankets occasionally made their way to Amara. Narrelle believed you could easily spot an Australian blanket, as they were particularly soft and woolly compared with the regular army blankets that were, Narrelle described, like coarse, heavy horse blankets.

Narrelle and the nursing staff were also given regular Hindustani lessons so that they could communicate with their patients, orderlies and camp followers who assisted with the running of the hospital. In her little black book, remnants of Narrelle's attempts at learning the language survive. She has lists of numbers, one to twenty; phrases such as 'light this', 'bring chair'; words for foods; and other useful phrases such as 'you son of a pig' and 'he is a great donkey'.

Although Narrelle's friend Jessie Stow was transferred to the smaller 23rd Stationary Hospital, positioned not far away from the river in the old Turkish quarters, there were a few Australian nurses to keep Narrelle company at the 32nd. Sister Jean Parker came from Queensland, had trained at the Sydney Hospital, and was engaged to one of the British officers on the river transports. Sister Weiss was from Melbourne, and Sister Annie Nelson hailed from South Australia. There were also Australian wireless squadrons in Mesopotamia and a group of pilots and mechanics sent by the Australian government to assist the campaign in early 1915. Called the Mesopotamian Half Flight, four pilots and fifty mechanics were seconded to the Mesopotamian campaign. Nine of the group were caught up in the Kut siege and were captured by the Turks, with seven later dying as POWs.

Narrelle bumped into Maurice Barton, a family friend, in April 1917. He had enlisted as a driver in the 1st Australian Wireless Squadron and left Australia in July 1916. A similar age to Narrelle, Maurice was married to Mabel, and lived in Leura in the Blue Mountains.

> *Maurice Barton, he came in another day to see me but I was awfully busy, and could only spare him a very few minutes. He said he would come in again before he left the Convalescent Camp, but I think he must have been switched back again to Baghdad, for he has not been over again. He said they were sending him back up the river. I should have liked to have seen him again before he went, you simply don't know the joy it was to sit there and just yap, to a really real man. The men stationed here, or the majority of them, remind me of soppy shop-walkers, and as for the majority of the women — Someone remarked one day that she had come to the conclusion that to be popular out here one must make one-self absolutely cheep* [sic] *especially with the men, so I just remarked that I was afraid the society of the majority of people out here troubled me so little, that I preferred unpopularity, to popularity on those terms.*
>
> *I like the man Parker is engaged to, he is rather a dear, but those women have utterly and absolutely spoilt the rest, or most of them. They lost their heads poor souls, when they were raised to the level — or rank — of an officer upon joining the QAIMNSR's for many of them have*

not an H in their dictionary. So there you have it — in a nutshell, and you can imagine how I am looking forward to my nice clean — keen Australians again.

Despite their remote location, the four Australian sisters received supplies from the Australian Comforts Fund's division in Melbourne. They were thrilled to receive one case of tomato soup, one case of tinned vegetables and one of tinned fruit — all hard to obtain, wonderful treats, and a variation from their largely dull and uneventful diet. So even though they, at times, felt disengaged from the world, the patriotic funds were a reminder that they were not forgotten by the Australian people. That meant a great deal. The funds also supplied cigarettes and tobacco. Most of the nurses, including Narrelle, were smokers. She liked nothing better than to sit down and smoke a cigarette. This habit was not mentioned in her letters until Mesopotamia so whether she picked up the habit on active service or was a smoker before the war is unclear. Her family and others sent her cigarettes as these, Narrelle said, were often unobtainable in Amara. *Let me add* she wrote, *smoking is a forbidden fruit, but — as an Englishman's house is his castle, so, an Australian's room is dashed well her own and the cigarettes in it — ah, I feel better now.*

Obtaining good supplies of clean water in Amara was always a challenge. The problem was that all water supplies — drinking water, washing, cleaning, and bathing — came from the one source — the Tigris River. The river was also used as a sewer and place to dump all manner of rubbish, so it was rather polluted. Chlorinating the water was generally the treatment of choice for authorities but this often made the tea undrinkable. Narrelle described how the *dhobi*, or washerman, laundered their clothes.

The river water is too awful for washing good things in, I always wash my own singlets, bloomers, hankies and collars for the Dhobie is too weird, and our beautiful white aprons, petticoats and overalls are a sort of dingy cream. You see the Dhobie (washerman) has a sort of landing stage of boards, built along the bank of the river, then he stands in the river and (damn cold these days) then he picks out an article of clothing from the bundle, dips it in the river and lathers it with soap, after which he proceeds to get the dirt out by doing physical exercises with his arms, the article of clothing being the dumbell, he twirls it airily round his head, and swish down it comes on to the boards, or, if they can get stones, all the better.

In Mesopotamia, the nurses still had the problem of hair loss. Whether it was the water, the general climate, or stress is unclear but Narrelle discussed the paltry state of everyone's hair quite often. Some of her colleagues were almost completely bald, she noted. Narrelle was very concerned and continued to use coconut oil and other concoctions on her hair. Whilst effective, they smelt awful, but she felt it was worth it as they gummed the hair to her scalp. She was afraid to wash her hair for fear it would simply all fall out. *I assure you, we are all most pathetic and have decided that the day we arrive in London we will make a bee line for a hair-dresser and try and get some locks.*

Later, she confided, *I'm now trying quinine and castor oil for my hair to see if that will stop it falling, for it's really getting quite distressing. I've fairly soaked it in cocoanut oil, certainly there are crowds of tiny hairs growing all through it, and it's fairly thick at the roots, but the back hair is scarcely any longer than the front hair now. It does not show under a cap, but heavens only knows how I shall ever do it when I get back to civilization.*

AFTER THE DISASTROUS BEGINNING TO THE MESOPOTAMIAN CAMPAIGN, culminating in the fall of Kut in April 1916, the British appointed the fresh-faced and relatively youthful Sir Frederick Maude to command the British forces. From July 1916, he re-organised the troops and military equipment, and revamped the transportation and medical facilities. One of the main problems with the earlier campaign was the sickness rate among reinforcements. Often troops became ill and were invalided back to India without firing a shot. This was in part due to the lack of suitable medical facilities, a problem which had been attended to, but also to the types of troops being sent to Mesopotamia. A committee established to investigate this issue recommended in July 1916 that young men under twenty and older recruits were unsuitable for Mesopotamia and should not be considered. The committee also recommended that all troops be sent to India for a time to acclimatise before being transported to Mesopotamia.

By October 1916, Maude had over 150,000 soldiers at his disposal in Mesopotamia as he prepared to retake Kut before the winter rains descended. Because of previous military failings, Maude needed permission from a sceptical war office in London to advance on Kut, 153 miles (245 kilometres) further up the Tigris River from Amara. However, Maude's organisation and leadership skills were impressive, and with all preparations in place, he was given the green light for an advance in December 1916. Maude and a force of 50,000 men attacked the Turks at Kut during the night of 13–14 December. By the end of January, the town had fallen to the British, and Maude, flushed with his successes, stormed on to Baghdad, which fell in March 1917.

Narrelle and her colleagues knew 'the push' was on from early December. Although work was always constant, with patients presenting with the usual range of illnesses such as dysentery, diarrhoea, and enteric fever, they were warned to prepare for a busy time ahead. Some nurses were transferred to convoy transports, which sailed up and down the river from Amara to the casualty clearing stations of Sheikh Saad, a journey that generally took two days. Whilst 'rushes' began, with convoys descending on the 32nd at frequent intervals, General Maude's campaign to retake Kut was delayed through bad weather. The winter rains, a feature of the region, began in early December, just as the campaign got underway. Narrelle described her first taste of the rain, and its immediate impact, to her family in a letter on 10 December.

The whole earth is turned into one large mud patch, mud, oh dear life, the black soil plains after two inches of rain are nothing to this, its such slippy mud, and so squidgy mud. You see we are built along the banks of the Tigris really, and this soil just sort of soaks up the water from the river, and right in our rooms and in the wards, the mud floors are simply soaking wet, and its soaking up the walls. I can see myself living in my gum boots and as they are fairly large I can get two pairs of stockings on. I'm bagging all the little chocks of wood I can to put under my trunk and kit bag, to keep them off the ground.

By early December it was also cold in Mesopotamia, in fact it was downright freezing at night. Narrelle received parcels from home with warm vests, bloomers and knitted spencers, a fabulous fur rug from Kit, and other essentials. Despite the cold, she was still sleeping outdoors, rather than in their 'matting enclosures' but she wore the following to bed: *I have a double blanket and a single, my warm nightie and a cotton kimino, long knitted bedsocks up over my knees and am not any too hot*. The nurses were issued with a grey woollen jumper that buttoned down the front to be worn after sunset. But Narrelle found the jumper so prickly and horrible that it gave her a heat rash around the neck and wrists, so she declined to wear it.

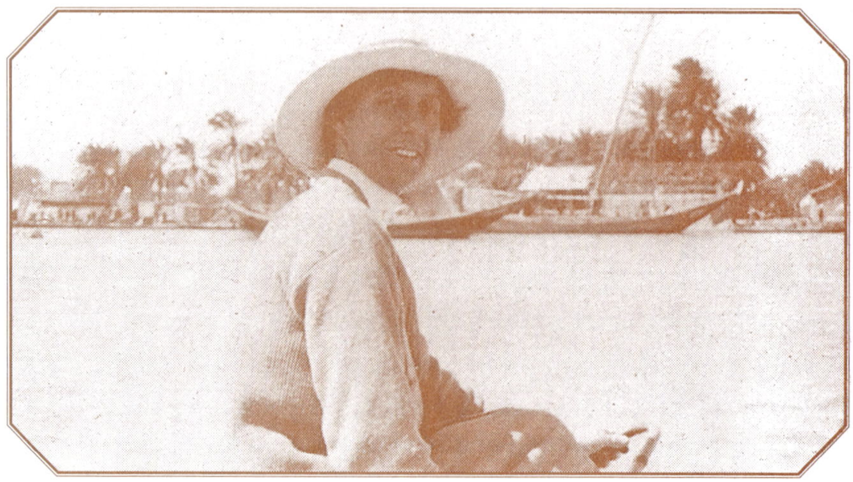

Boating on the Tigris River. Narrelle in Amara, 1917. (*Hobbes Collection*)

The weather had certainly turned. In the 32nd British General Hospital which hugged the river banks, it was cold, misty, wet, and very, very muddy. At night a dense fog would rise up from the river, blanketing the hospital in a veil of light mist-like rain. When the sun shone it was beautiful, but when it was cloudy and misty all day everything remained damp and wet to touch. Nurses tried to keep their huts warm and their patients comfortable, and keep out the chill winds and fog swirling around outside. Shutters were kept down along the huts to keep out the fog but it was hard to heat them when precious little supplies of coal or wood were available.

NARRELLE SPENT HER SECOND CHRISTMAS AWAY FROM AUSTRALIA, AND it was certainly different to her first one in Sicily. It was a time of reflection for all who found themselves so far from home. She longed for peace and to return home to her beloved family. She had had enough. Sometimes she wondered if it would ever end, if she would ever return to a normal life. Indeed, she sometimes believed that this strange military existence she was leading, in a land far away, was how things were going to be for evermore.

In an effort to create some Christmas cheer for the patients and staff alike, the sisters were given an allowance from Matron Jones to decorate their wards. Narrelle used date palm leaves and small clay water holders, called 'chatties', which came in all shapes and sizes and were, most importantly, cheap to buy in the markets. She purchased coloured paper and coloured muslin and, attached to twigs from pomegranate trees, made a 'garden' of sweet peas. Arches of palm leaves were tied to the ward posts, and Narrelle managed to borrow three flags to which she added her small Australian one. Narrelle's ward, Hut No 3, was voted the prettiest, of course. On Christmas Eve, in the evening, one of the medical officers dressed up as Santa Claus and, with Matron Jones and the sisters, distributed presents to the patients. Later, Narrelle joined a group that went round singing carols accompanied by string instruments played by orderlies, the padre, quartermaster, and a patient playing a little tiny organ.

On Christmas Day, Narrelle made a trifle from two Swallow and Ariel sponge cakes for her 'on diet' patients and procured jelly, a rare treat, for the 'no diet' patients. So that everyone could have an enjoyable Christmas, staff were rostered to work either Christmas or Boxing Day, with the other day off. Narrelle worked on the 25th and therefore had her Christmas dinner on Boxing Day. It consisted of roast wild goose, plum pudding, wine, crackers and sweets brought up by Matron Beatrice Jones from Bombay months before. It was these sorts of gestures and the thought that went into them that made Beatrice Jones so well liked and well respected by her staff. After singing carols, about 26 of the group headed across the river to the YMCA hut to see the

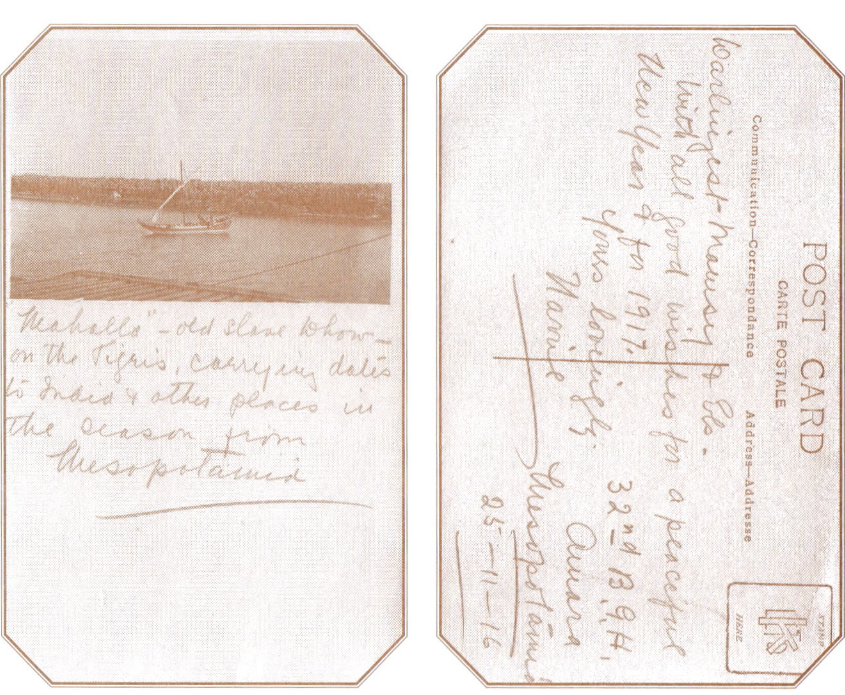

Another of Narrelle's photographs made into a postcard, this time Christmas and New Year greetings. (*Hobbes Collection*)

1916 silent, black and white movie *When Knights were Bold*, by British director Maurice Elvey. The weather was atrocious. It poured with rain, so Narrelle donned her raincoat, sou'wester, and gumboots. With her dress pinned up over her knees, she headed off into the darkness, praying that she would not slip over in the greasy, sticky mud. It was a memorable Christmas, certainly more enjoyable than her 1915 one in Sicily. Where, Narrelle wondered, would she spend her next one?

WITH THE CAMPAIGN STILL UNDERWAY IN THE FIRST MONTHS OF 1917, the convoys of wounded and sick patients continued to arrive. The soldiers had various nicknames for their injuries and illnesses. Slight wounds were called a 'Basra' wound, more serious ones were an 'India' wound; and 'Blighty' meant a significant, usually long-term recovery, with possible medical discharge in England. Narrelle learnt that 'Blighty' was the British soldier's interpretation of *bilate*, the Hindustani term for 'across the sea'. Alternatively if the soldier's wounds only rated a 'CD' (Convalescent Depot), that meant rest and recuperation in Mesopotamia. According to Narrelle, an enteric patient was *always* "*India*". Often the nursing staff had very little notice of impending arrivals, as Narrelle related cheerily in a letter home on Tuesday, 30 January 1917.

> *Ye gods, talk about our first days in Malta, hum, I started this letter on Friday, with nothing to do, just filling in time, no, it was Saturday evening. I had 14 patients in my ward and had lent all my sisters but one, to the huts where they were busy. Went on duty next morning at 7.30, just as the convoy bugle went, and before I knew where I was, 45 of my beds were filled up, and I couldn't get another sister.*
>
> *Work? This is the first time I've got off duty since, except for meals, and now, just as I've got hold of my pad, there is that convoy bugle again, and I must go on, for I've only left one sister on duty and if we get another rush, for I've still got a good many beds, it's too much for one.*

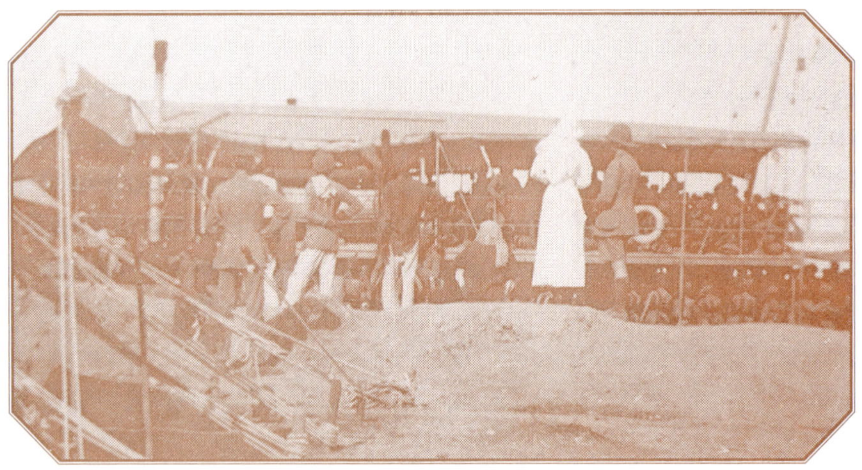

Embarking the wounded for Basra, 1917. (*Hobbes Collection*)

> *Today I've got another Australian girl with me, a Miss Parker, Queensland but was trained at the 'Sydney' and she is on duty alone, she is such a dear — the unfortunate theatre people are going like slaves, two theatres, the men are most cheerful tho, and oh I do like surgical work, it's the joke of the Hospital that poor old Hut 3 (mine) is turned into a surgical ward for all its life, been Enteric, but we have no Enterics, or only three or four, so — Adieu.*

Baghdad was occupied in March 1917 and the medical infrastructure soon followed. Nurses did not particularly want to be transferred to Baghdad; they believed it to be hotter and less clean than Amara. Nevertheless, Jessie Stow and the 23rd Stationary Hospital moved there in May 1917, taking over the Turkish Military Hospital. It took considerable time to fumigate and clean the hospital, which was in a pitiable state, but soon there was an isolation hospital, an officers' convalescent depot and an officers' hospital in operation. Narrelle's friend Colonel Thomas Legg also kept in touch, writing regularly. He was posted to Shiekh Saad further up the river from Amara, where he suffered from hay fever due to the dust. Like Jessie Stow, he was later transferred to Baghdad.

During the first months of 1917, life in Amara at the 32nd British General Hospital was a mixture of work and play. Whilst there were limited recreational activities, apart from the pictures at the YMCA or playing sporting games, Narrelle did enjoy wandering through Amara, and going to the bazaars to pick up some souvenirs and presents. She explained to her family the art of bartering in a letter from 17 January 1917.

> *The usual method when buying anything is to go to the shop, which is just a little 5 by 5 hollow on the street somewhere. Inside are the owners, sitting cross legged on the floor. If it's a silversmith, he and his son or*

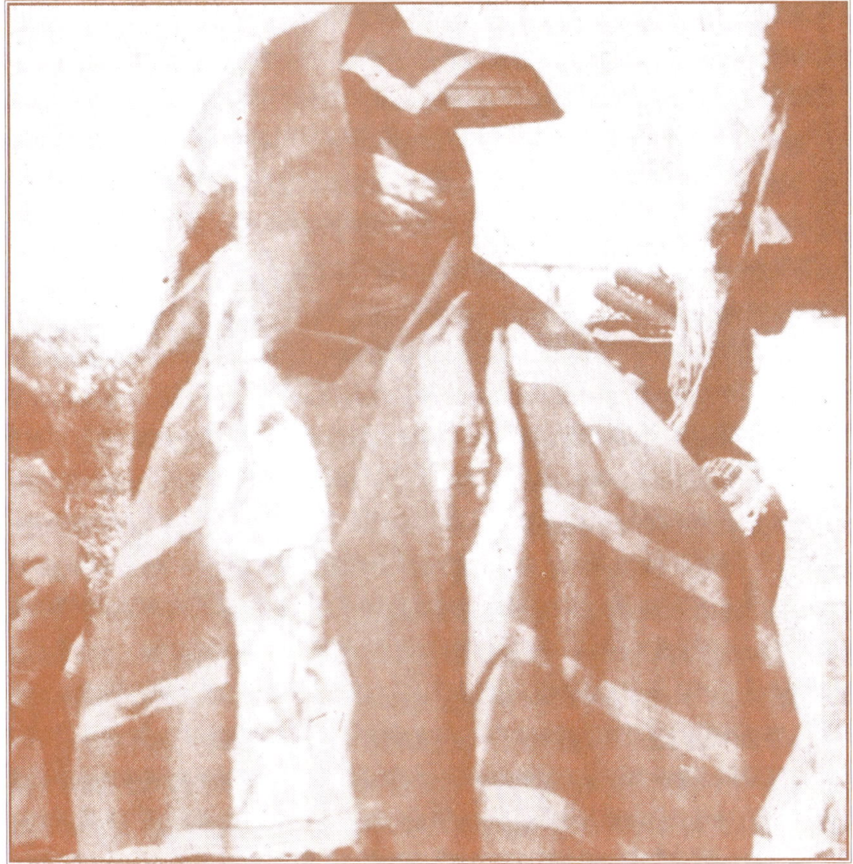

Arab woman in Amara, 1917. (*Hobbes Collection*)

partner will be working away at some work, with a tiny fire in a hollowed out stone nearby. You sit down on the step, which is about a foot or two feet high, or on a little flat stool just inside the shop and casually pick up some article, say in a bored way 'Aysh qimat hatha?' 'What is the price of this?' and they will say some absurd price three times what it is worth so you say 'La' 'No' and so it goes on, you sit on looking at things in a bored way and he will come down a Rupee but that is not enough so once more you say 'La' you have said Rupee 5, and it you sit stolidly on, he will continue to come down, one rupee at a time, and at last will take up the article and put it in your hand 'Take it' and you ask 'Rupee 5?' and it is yours, but sometimes it is necessary to get up and walk away, but some of them are so independent that not even that will help you, so you do without — for it's absurd and not right, to give what they ask. Some of the sisters and officers give them any bally old thing they ask for, and then they simply won't sell for anything under, it's so silly and wrong really, for these Arabs, and the Indians too, are brought up from their earliest infancy to <u>*do*</u> *less cunning people, people who have not the placid philosophy to sit out a bargain as their own people will, they really are quite fascinating in their philosophical outlook.*

By April 1917, the rain, mud and fog were replaced by rising temperatures and an invasion of insects. Despite being issued with mosquito nets, Narrelle described an appalling night of sandflies, mosquitoes, fleas, *and millions of other insects crawling over you, biting you and tearing the very flesh off in strips*. Sleep was almost impossible. As the temperatures rose, the dust storms came, which created more challenges. Narrelle always compared the differing climatic changes with Cobar or Brewarrina. She might have complained about Malta, Sicily and Bombay, but Mesopotamia was unique in its intensity and ferocity. Everything was magnified. She had never encountered such a raging and inhospitable climate. She wrote home on 3 May in the middle of a furious dust storm. As she wrote, perspiration was trickling down her back, neck, breasts and stomach in a constant steady stream.

Oh my beloveds,

If you could see me now, never in Cobar or Brewarrina's wildest summer moments could they ever reach anything like this, gee whiz, as I write mounds of dust are forming on my papers. In fact I've almost to dig my way through to get to the paper at all, and every spot is simply inches deep with it. The patients look like red plasticine objects in bed, and you can hardly see from one end of the hut to the other, and figures moving about, mist of fine grey dust, never, never have I seen anything like it, and it's been doing this for three days and nights, and you have probably observed in Reuters that 'Progress in Mesopotamia was hindered by dust storms'.

Last night when I undressed, through to my very skin was soft fine grey powder, and all the seams of my underclothes were marked with it, you eat it, you breathe it, you drink it, and you should see the way it has gathered along the hinge of this paper, gosh I can hardly see out of my eyes, and I want to sneeze my head off ... fortunately I've never had it [hay fever] *since I left Australia, but if this dust keeps up for many more days, I can see myself retiring from active service with the Adrenalin bottle.*

IT WAS NOW JUNE 1917. NARRELLE HAD BEEN WORKING IN MESOPOTAMIA since September the previous year without a break. That was nine months' continuous active service in one of the most challenging and physically demanding theatres of World War I. All up, she had endured two years on active service without a proper break. Whilst she was talking to her family about taking leave in either the Himalayas or England later in the year, nothing was official. She did consider resigning from the QAIMNS but, if she did, she would have to make her own way back home, something that was unthinkable for her. It would be giving up. And, in any event, she could not afford the fare. It was too expensive.

Matron Beatrice Jones was acutely aware of the pressures placed on her staff and the physical toll the extreme conditions were taking on them. From December 1916 to September 1917 almost 100 nurses were evacuated to India from illness, mainly dysentery, enteric fever and malaria. Hundreds more were hospitalised in sickbay for various minor conditions such as heat stroke. Matron Jones, too, was fully aware that sisters like Narrelle had had no leave and were long overdue for some rest and recreation. In order for nurses to take leave, however, there needed to be sufficient replacements, and there was a general scarcity of nurses willing to serve in Mesopotamia. However, eventually Matron Jones informed Narrelle that she would be given leave in July. Sisters who had been in Malta and Egypt took preference over those who had come out straight from England.

Narrelle never took her leave. Instead, she succumbed to illness, an abhorrent state for any nurse. Sick sisters were *looked on as a bore,* Narrelle later wrote to her family. They were there to heal and make soldiers well, not to fall sick themselves. Narrelle had a robust constitution and had not been seriously ill during the two years she had been on active service. Despite some weight and hair loss and other minor complaints along the way, she had kept reasonably healthy with her iron tonics and regular dosages of cod liver oil. Being a nurse, she knew how to look after herself. But the lack of leave and respite from her war nursing eventually took its toll.

One evening, in early June 1917, just after she had come off duty, Narrelle's face suddenly swelled up with dark red welts around it. She felt nauseous and vomited throughout the night. The following day, Matron sent her to sickbay with *contusion of face* and a slight temperature. As she explained to her family:

> *I used to be allowed up for two or three hours after sunset, and generally went for a walk on the river but always felt deadly seedy when up, then the heat was so awful, 124* [degrees] *and so hot that you could hardly stand it. I used to fairly shake my fist at the sun, and swear at it, it seemed to fairly gloat over us, and dance for joy, oh it was dreadful. I had a punka over my bed but could only keep it just moving, otherwise the air*

came down so hot on me, that it fairly burnt me. How the men stood it, left in the trenches, and doing fatigue work, I simply don't know.

She was in sickbay for a week but, rather than recovering, became steadily worse. Her eyes began to go yellow (a sign of jaundice) so it was decided to send her to Bombay with the next hospital convoy. Jaundice was particularly prevalent in the summer months in Mesopotamia, and it was the most common illness after diarrhoea, enteric fever and malaria. In tropical countries jaundice can be associated with malaria, or hepatitis transmitted through contaminated food or water, or it can be a symptom of a tumour in the liver, bile duct system or pancreas. Jaundice required specialist treatment not available in Mesopotamia.

During World War I significant advances were made in the diagnosis and treatment of jaundice. It was found that rat's urine contaminated water and food, which explained the epidemic of jaundice that occurred in the trenches on the western front among French, German and British troops. Symptoms included high fever, headache and body pains, vomiting, diarrhoea, enlargement of the liver, and haemorrhages. Recovery was slow but generally the disease was not fatal.

The next medical convoy was leaving Amara immediately. Narrelle had only two hours' notice to pack up all her things and to say her goodbyes. She was feeling dreadful so was placed on a stretcher and carried onto the riverboat, and into a tiny, hot, stifling cabin. Despite feeling awfully sick, she managed to drag herself out onto the deck to watch the magnificent sunset across the shimmering desert reflected in the waters of the Euphrates and Tigris rivers. It was the last Mesopotamian sunset Narrelle would see. She became so unwell that she remained inside her cabin for the rest of the journey. The convoy arrived at Basra at night, and Narrelle was carried on a stretcher on the shoulders of four men to the No 3 British General Hospital. After nine months, she was back again but this time she was a patient not a nurse.

Narrelle found herself in a ward with sixteen other sick sisters, all admitted for sandfly fever, another prevalent disease in the summer months. Caused by the bite of the insect, the symptoms included a raging temperature and extreme vomiting. However, this illness was not considered serious enough to warrant a trip to Bombay. Narrelle's condition, on the other hand, was a different matter. By this stage she was turning a strange shade of yellow all over her body, and was earmarked for immediate evacuation to Bombay on the next available hospital ship. As she related to her family:

> *I began to feel more particularly rotten: and began to turn a most beautiful colour, it would have made any canary turn green with envy, as it was I began to turn a beautiful yellow green, like nothing on earth or in the sea. I absolutely could not bear to look at my own face in the glass, from the crown of my head to the tip of my toes, you can't imagine just how beautiful I looked, and gosh didn't I feel rotten.*

After a week of waiting, Narrelle left Basra on 17 June, and embarked on the hospital ship *Eranpura*. Her slow journey continued down the Shatt-el-Arab. The searing heat was almost too much for her. As she explained:

> *... oh, the heat, great shade of Omar, the heat I thought my body would just surely burst with the heat. I didn't know how to lie, sit or stand, every spot was absolutely red and to make matters worse, we had to wait inside the river till next morning, as we had just missed the tide across the bar. There wasn't a breath of air, and the heat was too awful for words, you know when you can't get away from things, and your very eyeballs perspire and you feel that if you don't get some air, or the sun doesn't go down, you will just expire. All that night was like a refined form of torture.*

Finally, they crossed the bar and were ferried out to the *Herefordshire*, a hospital ship staffed by Australian nurses. Though weak and unable to walk, she was thrilled to be nursed by her compatriots, all from

Melbourne. It was smooth sailing but once they got around the Strait of Harmutz and out into the Gulf of Oman, the monsoon struck. They sailed slowly and carefully along the coast to Karachi where 200 Indian invalids were disembarked, but were then hit by the full force of the monsoon and chaos reigned for five days. Almost all the nursing staff and crew were seasick. Narrelle was surrounded with pillows, tightly packed in so that she would not fall out of her berth. Everything lurched from side to side, and the ship rolled around so much that Narrelle heard items being thrown about and crockery smashing throughout the ship. It was a horrendous passage. On reaching Bombay, Narrelle learnt of the sinking of the *Mongolia*, a P & O passenger ship, which had been only 15 miles (24 kilometres) ahead of them. The ship hit a mine and the explosion destroyed the wireless, so no SOS was sent out. The survivors included three Australian nursing sisters on their way back to Melbourne.

Narrelle was admitted to the Colaba War Hospital. She could not believe it. Almost exactly a year on, she was back in Bombay, in the middle of the dreaded monsoon. Only this time she was very ill.

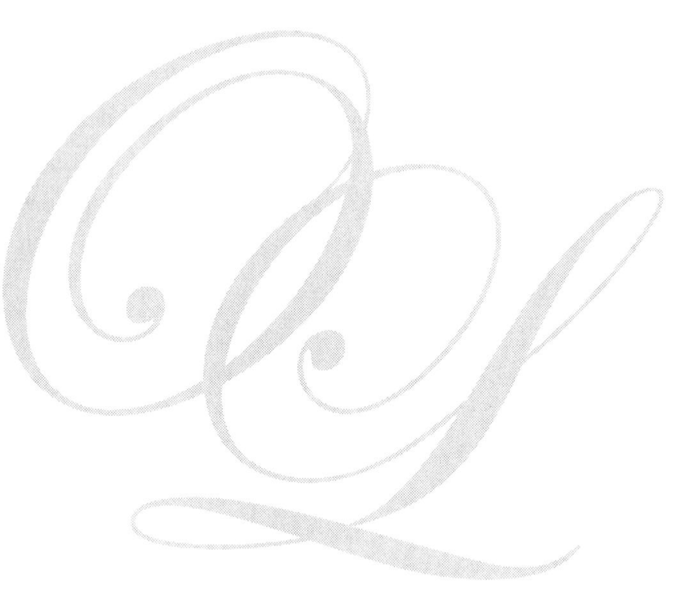

THE HIMALAYAS

Chapter 9

'HOWLING LIKE A FROSTBITTEN DINGO'

THERE WAS A FLURRY OF ACTIVITY AT 'BALBLAIR', MRS HOBBES' HOUSE in Cremorne. A cablegram had just been delivered. It came from the War Office in London. Elsie Hobbes ran through the house looking for her mother. A wave of panic swept over her; the telegram had to be about Narrelle. Her mother was out in the garden tending to her roses. Elsie handed her the telegram in silence. Margaret Hobbes swapped the secateurs for the cream envelope, and opened it in one swift movement, her nails ripping the envelope into two pieces in her haste.

The cable was a really an official typed 'form letter' with spaces left for information concerning a specific soldier or nurse. The large cursive handwriting was commanding, pressing into the paper, certainly a male hand. It was dated 21 June 1917. Margaret Hobbes read its contents aloud to Elsie.

> *The Military Secretary presents his compliments to Mrs Hobbes and begs to inform her that the following report has just been received from the Embarkation Commandant Basra dated June 17th Sister N. Hobbes was Invalided to India, for Bombay. Further reports will be sent when received.*

A second cablegram was received the following week. Dated 24 June and sent from Karachi in India, it stated that Narrelle had arrived there safely, and was re-embarked for Bombay, suffering from jaundice. Her condition was favourable. A third cable was despatched to Mrs Hobbes on 1 July 1917, informing her that her daughter was admitted to the Colaba War Hospital, Bombay.

COLABA WAR HOSPITAL WAS A LARGE RAMBLING INSTITUTION ON THE outskirts of Bombay, staffed by Australian and British nurses from the AANS and QAIMNS. There were also English VADs and RAMC orderlies, as well as many Indian orderlies and helpers. The hospital incorporated 100 beds for British officers, 500 beds for other ranks, a smaller sisters' hospital, and special wards for dysentery and malaria patients.

Narrelle was admitted to the Sick Sisters' Hospital and within two weeks she was feeling better. Her temperature returned to normal and she lost the deep sickly yellow tinge of jaundice. She also gained weight. Even though she did not feel exactly 100 per cent, she was busting to get out of hospital. Narrelle wanted to escape Bombay with its dreaded monsoon and blistering heat. It was not her favourite place. She busied herself planning her convalescent leave, where she would go and what she might do. But first she had to pass an examination by the medical board, or, as she referred to it, her 'board'. This was where the military medical authorities assessed the health and wellbeing of a patient, to decide whether the nurse or soldier was fit again for active service, required more leave, had to be invalided back to England for extended leave or specialist treatment, or, in extreme circumstances, be discharged from the army.

It was decided by the board that Narrelle was to have a month's recuperation up in the cool and refreshing Himalayas, at one of the hill stations of her choice. Narrelle was keen to go somewhere small, certainly not to the popular spots of Simla or Darjeeling where thousands regularly sought refuge from the heat of the Indian summer.

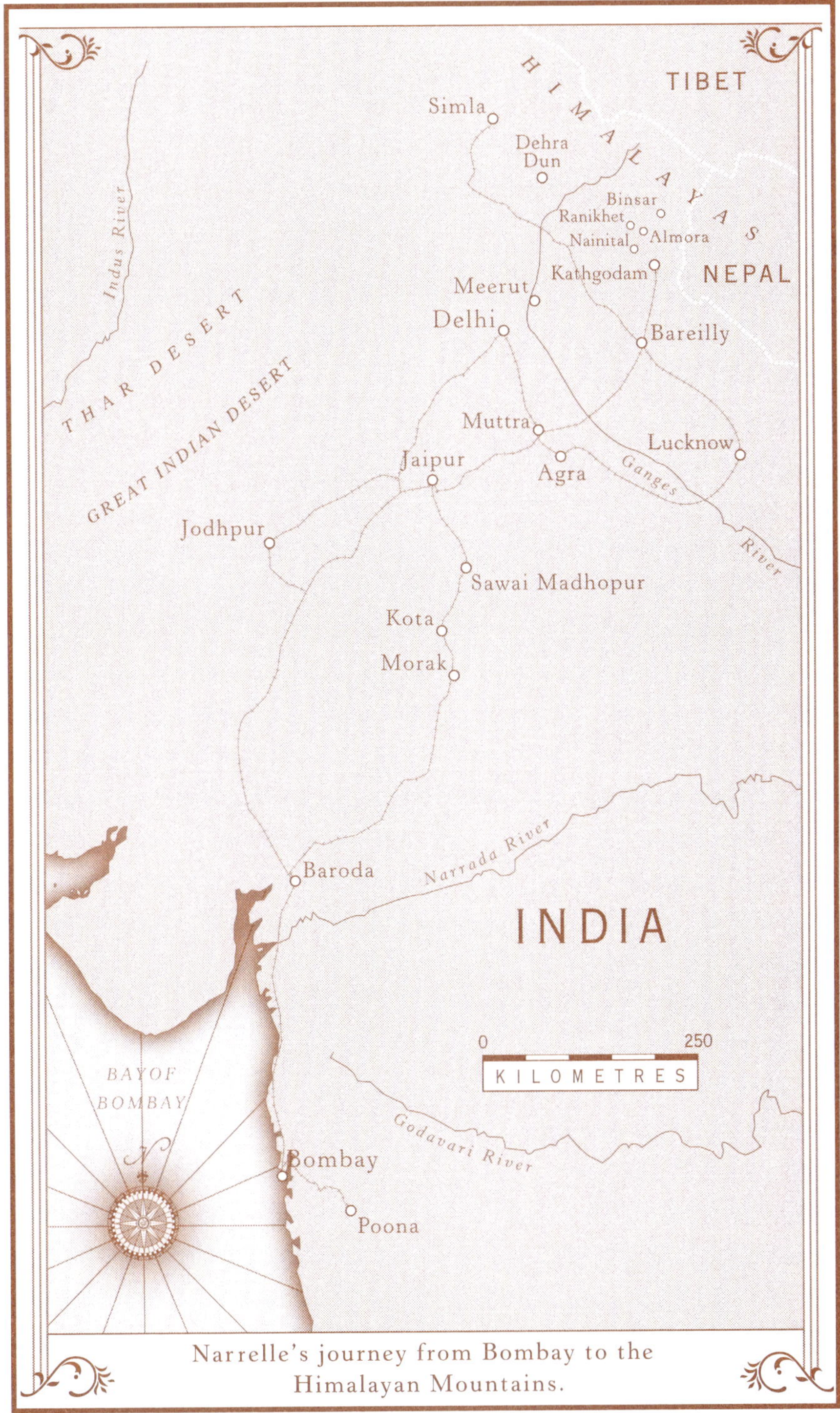

Narrelle's journey from Bombay to the Himalayan Mountains.

She wanted somewhere off the beaten track, somewhere a little more interesting, somewhere less touristy. Most importantly, because money was always tight, she wanted to go somewhere cheap.

Narrelle chose Binsar, an isolated hill station in the foothills of the Himalayas near Almora, which in 1917 was inaccessible by road. Even today Binsar is a remote wildlife sanctuary and national park, well known for its forests of Himalayan oaks, deodars and rhododendrons. There is an abundance of wonderful bird life, such as whistling thrushes, scarlet minarets and owlets, as well as leopards, deer and wild boars. To get to Binsar from Bombay, a distance of almost 1000 miles (1600 kilometres), Narrelle would have to journey by train across the Indian subcontinent as far as Kathgodam, the end of the line. She then would have to travel to Almora and Binsar by other means. Just getting to her hill station was going to be an adventure.

Narrelle was granted leave until 12 September, which was exactly three months from the day she was invalided back to Bombay from Basra. It was common practice to give nurses three months' sick leave. After her accommodation and pay was organised, and the authorities had prepared transport papers and warrant passes, she was a 'free woman'. Allowed to travel in mufti, a state she had not experienced for almost a year, Narrelle headed off on her sick leave. To make sure her family was not worrying unnecessarily, she sent a cablegram to her mother reassuring the family that she had recovered and that she was heading for the Himalayas for some well-earned leave.

But Narrelle did not tell them of her stomach pains. As she was about to be discharged from the hospital, Narrelle felt terrible pains in her abdomen. She described them as a *beastly indigestion sort of pain*. Three times she mentioned it to a medical officer at the Colaba War Hospital. As she later told her family, he *didn't think anything of it, said with his idiotic & inane laugh which used to make us think he wasn't all there, 'Oh yes, you'll get rid of that as you get stronger' & gave me Bismuth and Mist to take*. Bismuth and Mist was a general medicine used to treat indigestion, nausea, stomach cramps and diarrhoea. Narrelle, being Narrelle, did not make too much of it. She was the stoic type. She was not going to let intermittent stomach pains interrupt her holiday plans, particularly if it meant staying any longer in Bombay, so she did not push it further. One can only speculate what the medical authorities were doing allowing a nurse to leave their care, to discharge her, without ensuring that she had returned to full health. This was to be a fatal mistake.

Narrelle did not make a fuss for another reason. How could her minor illness compare with what the boys were going through in Mesopotamia, Egypt, and on the western front? The day she left Bombay Narrelle received word that her cousin Gilbert Anschau, whom she had last seen in Malta two years earlier, was wounded and missing in action in France. Due to the lack of news, and because she had been ill, Narrelle had not heard about the raging battles on the western front during the spring of 1917 involving Australian troops. Narrelle was shocked at the report. Those three words cast a long, dark shadow over her. She knew what 'wounded and missing' really meant.

> *Poor Gilbert, when I hear of them being wounded & missing it makes a coward of me. When I think of the stories my patients have told me re the fate of those wounded & unable to get back from 'No Man's Land' & I can only say God help those dear men & out of their misery quickly, it's too awful, poor dear souls, & I do sincerely hope Gilbert has been able to get back to our lines, or been taken prisoner, tho the latter would be a hateful fate for him, poor boy.*

Sadly, as described earlier, Gilbert Anschau was confirmed killed on 17 September 1917, his body never found. So it was with a heavy heart that Narrelle put her 'minor' stomach complaint to one side and, in the first week of August 1917, left Bombay. Narrelle described her lengthy, tiring but immensely fascinating train journey across the heart of India in great detail to her family. Anyone who has experienced Indian train travel will agree that it is an unforgettable adventure. The chaotic nature of the train stations and the sheer numbers of people travelling en masse, as if the whole of India is on the move at the one time, combined with the uniquely Indian way of doing things remain etched in the traveller's memory forever.

Class and race were, and still are, keenly noted when travelling by train in India. The trains had first, second and third class carriages, and people were segregated according to their race, caste and gender. Narrelle shared a first class carriage with an English VAD who was travelling to Muttra (present day Mathura) on the Yamuna River, the reputed birth-place of the Hindu god Krishna. There were also eight British officers on the train, along with hundreds and hundreds of Indian passengers. As Narrelle explained to her family, she was told to travel light, so her luggage was a tiffin basket:

> *...containing thermos, Tommy Cooker (do you know what that is? It's a tin containing solid methylated, a wee stand, tiny dixey and a tin of refill) some biscuits, the milk, tea and other things out of your last parcel, & some books (many thanks for that parcel dears all ...) medicine & a few odds & ends. Then another basket (they are square, strongly made with round cane), filled with clothing, not a very large one, my suitcase, & hold all the latter holding my boots, polishing things, possum rug, blanket, coat, sheets & pillow. These things all quite necessary when travelling in India, for even in the best hotels they never supply you with blankets, & often not even with sheets, oh my dears it's the very quaintest place possible! There are no lavatories outside Bombay, simply a bathroom attached to your room & in that a commode, but, every bedroom has its own bathroom & very often dressing room attached, so well to continue, you also mostly have to take your own lav paper, truly, out of the towns, it's a most primitive place.*

Narrelle's carriage was spacious. It was:

> *... as large as a room, with whole bathroom attached, this was reserved for we two nurses, they have tremendously wide gauge on all the long*

distance trainways here, the seats pulled out to the width of a wide single bed, & there was room for all our luggage without it taking up any room, so it seemed, for as well as my four things.

We had to go through some of the most utterly & absolutely filthy places, slums of Bombay, that fairly stank again, til we got to a place called Viar, then the country began to open out & was rather beautiful, numbers of paddy fields, & green grass, oh, the green ness of everything during the rains in India, it's wonderful, then towards sunset we began to come to water, it looked like a huge river till we got to it, & discovered it was the arm of the sea that turns Bombay into an island, and there is a most wonderful bridge over it, a mile long, it has no side arches or railing, just bridge. We had to go very slowly over it, & by the time we got on to the other side, the dusk had settled down & we made up our beds, & after supper went to bed, but somehow I could not sleep, & when we stopped at the various stations there was always the most unearthly noise with the swarms & swarms of yelling natives, the platform used to seem packed with them, all yelling at one another & fearfully excited, sleep was quite out of the question as long as you were at the station, however, after a bit, towards morning, I did go to sleep & was wakened about 7am by a voice at my shutter 'Chota Hazri Mem Sahib?' & tea was brought along.

The train's destination of Muttra was a distance of well over 600 miles (960 kilometres) to the north-east. As night fell, the train travelled north along the coast until Baroda (or Vadodara) and then turned inland, crossing the Malwa Plateau, and to the plains of Rajasthan.

We were now getting along into the plains of Central India … It made me quite homesick, positively, crossing those plains of Central India, it was most absurdly like Australia. First it was just like Bre country in a very good season, then it got sort of red hilly country like Cobar, it was continually changing. After a while it got rather like the country round Breeza, or higher up with small mountains in the distance, but all in a wonderfully good season, with mimosa trees & little strange clusters of bushes all about, but instead of sheep there were goats, and instead of our clean, straight backed cattle, mobs of strange looking hump backed animals & water buffalo, with their long evil Hippotamus faces & black hair, so short & sleek, that it looks like the skin of an elephant that has just come out of water, camels, wild peacocks, pigeons & always, always the ubiquitous native, with simply a loin cloth & old rag coat, or a native woman in brilliant hued clothes draped around her.

Narrelle felt the country near the small town of Morak, to the south of Kota in Rajasthan was *more Australian than anything I've seen for the last 2 & a half years, even to the occasional shiny leafed box tree, at least it looks like box, & grass, phew what grass, almost up to your waist. I felt as though I had just wakened up & found myself on the way to Bre or Warialda, oh dear, if it was only true with the war a thing of the past.*

Watching this scenery from her window, waves of homesickness crashed uncontrollably over her. As she sat with her elbow resting on the grimy windowsill, slowly caressed by the gentle rhythmic rocking of the train, Narrelle cried. Careful not to draw attention to herself, she kept her face turned toward the window, and quietly brushed away the hot tears. She could not stop thinking about Gilbert, Wilfred, Ted and Geoff Yeomans. Now four of her friends were dead. She was so out of touch in far away India that more of them could be dead or missing or seriously wounded and she would never know. She had not heard from any of the boys for a while, the mail was sporadic and unreliable. She felt completely alone in a country of 300 million people.

IT WAS POURING WITH RAIN AS THE TRAIN SLOWLY PULLED INTO SAWAI Madhopur station. It was one o'clock in the afternoon, lunchtime. Everyone piled off the train and the group of British officers and nurses were informed by an excitable stationmaster that the train line ahead was washed out and they had best return to Bombay and catch another train via Ahmadabad which went through central Rajasthan to Jaipur. Not keen to retrace her steps, Narrelle spent time poring over the largely incomprehensible Indian railway timetable and, after more discussions with the highly strung stationmaster, a second option to travel to Jaipur on the 5pm train, and from there connect to Mattra emerged. After a twelve-hour wait at Mattra, she could then catch the night train to Kathgodam. To Narrelle's relief, one of the British officers, the elderly Colonel Carruthers, who had recently spent six months in Australia and New Zealand, announced that he was travelling on in her direction, so they teamed up.

They arrived in Jaipur, the capital of Rajasthan, at 10.30 at night, dead tired and ready for bed. But after further consultation with timetables, they discovered that an overnight train to Agra was leaving immediately, from where they could make the connection to Kathgodam. After realising that the ladies carriage was full of Indian women and their children, *of course I could not possibly go in there, it was unheard of, for native & English women to herd together on the railway*, Narrelle took the more socially acceptable option of sharing a carriage with Colonel Carruthers. After enduring a painfully slow and tedious journey, they reached Agra mid-morning on Monday, 7 August.

Narrelle could not believe her luck. Thanks to the vagaries of the Indian railways and the weather, she found herself in Agra, home of the Taj Mahal, one of the most famous love shrines in the world. She was entranced from the moment the train pulled into the station just under the ancient brown walls of the old fort built by the Mogul emperor Akbar around 1565. With Colonel Carruthers in tow, Narrelle went straight to Laurie's Hotel, a colonial-designed hotel set on 15 acres of lawns and gardens about a mile from the station. It was far too hot to do any sightseeing so Narrelle had a bath, changed into fresh clothes, lunched and rested, with an Indian woman pulling a punka above her for some respite from the heat. At 3.30 in the afternoon, as it was getting slightly cooler, Colonel Carruthers and Narrelle

… got a carriage & pair, frightfully swanky, & went 3 miles out to see the Taj Mahal. Truly is it called the incomparable Taj Mahal, one of the seven wonders of the world, built by Shah Jahan, the luxurious, over the grave of his favourite wife, she was a Hindu. It's a pure white marble tomb, like a large house, with wonderful domes & spires, & it's so white that no birds will settle on it, on each side, there is a mosque. Inside there is a most wonderful echo, an old Indian will sing three notes, & it goes round & round getting fainter & fainter, then we went down to where the actual grave is, the old chappie got himself buried next to her, so the tomb does for them both, it was as cold as anything down there … it's a most beautiful sight, & the beautiful old gates, huge things, with wonderful designs & carvings on them, you sort of suddenly come onto them in the trees …

After the Taj Mahal, Narrelle and the colonel climbed back into their carriage and drove along the Yamuna River to the old fort, through the Delhi gate, and across an old drawbridge. Narrelle loved the Motif Masjid, or 'Pearl Mosque', built by Shah Jahan from 1646 to 1653. She described it to her family.

Right in the middle of the fort is the most beautiful Mosque I've ever seen, it's said to be the most beautiful in India. It has the most magnificent carved arches of marble, most exquisite carved, sort of fretwork doors, carved out of one block of marble, & every worshipper had a marble slab in place of a prayer mat, with a verse from the Koran on it — no, wait a minute, I think I'm wrong about the verse on each slab, it's another place that has that — but to stand at one side & look along those exquisitely carved pillars and arches, & the exquisite designs of those side doors, was a sight for the Gods, truly magnificent & then, in imagination, I filled it with worshippers, chanting in low, soft voices their beloved prayers, & verses from the Koran, & every now & again bowing their foreheads to the west, murmuring 'Allah is God, there is no God but god', oh it was all very great & wonderful, the Unchanging East … We went up into one of the domes, & looked out over Agra ... ah it was most beautiful the sun was just getting fairly low down and casting the softest lights & shades everywhere.

Narrelle and the colonel spent nearly two hours wandering through the fort admiring the Hindu architecture, the carved walls with elephants, little balconies with carved lattice work and marble railings. Before long it was time to head back to the train station to connect with their 7pm train, and the next phase of their journey. With their luggage already sent from the hotel, they found their respective carriages and settled in for the night train, two very tired but contented travellers. Overnight the train crossed the Ganges Delta, and sunrise saw it at Bareilly, a large town in Uttar Pradesh. The heat was oppressive, so Narrelle sat back in her carriage with two fans turned on full blast and the shutters closed on the eastern side.

On & on we went, along just a single line, through tropical trees and undergrowth, with swarms of little monkeys skipping along the ground whenever it was clear, & swinging up into the trees, oh the quaintest little things, all the time the heat was tremendous, hot & steamy, & bright sun, I began to wonder <u>when</u> it was going to start & get cool, suddenly away in the distance, we saw the mountains, the first edge of the Himalayas wrapped in cloud & purple mist, sending out a premise of coolth, we felt like the Greeks when they found the sea & cried 'Thalassa', ah! we breathe again in anticipation of it all, and can almost feel the coolness of the snows — in imagination, but it's another hour & half yet before we get to the funny little place called Kathgodam, the end of the railway, & we have to get out.

At Kathgodam, Narrelle farewelled the colonel, and set off by car with another British officer to Nainital. The winding road cut into the mountains and dropped away steeply on the other side through jungle filled with exquisitely coloured butterflies. They climbed over 4200 feet

(1280 metres) in 12 miles (19 kilometres), and reached the Brewery, a large whisky distillery and brewery established in the 1870s. It produced, Narrelle declared, the worst beer in India, but there was a good restaurant and place to stay if required. After a short rest, Narrelle embarked on the next phase of her journey to Nainital, Almora and Binsar, by *dandi*, a sedan chair carried by four *dandi-wallahs*, or *dandi-carriers*. This was a standard method of travel in the mountains for the British. As Narrelle explained:

> *At last we got to the Brewery, & shed the motor. We were at once surrounded by hordes of coolies with dandies, ponys & luggage coolies. The Officer man had his own, they had come down from Naini Tal for him. At last I got my dandi, which, let me here add is a boat shaped chair, with poles, carried on the shoulders of four coolies (provided they are not Brahmas. If they are, then you are carried on their heads, for a Brahman will not carry things on his shoulder) the dandi … has a hood generally, because of the sudden rains. It's a most quaint sensation when you first start, & if going up a steep place, you are carried up backwards, away down on one side. The road suddenly gives, & in places, especially during the rains, the road has been washed away, but the sure footed coolies know just how to carry you & the dandi never slips, up, up, up.*

It was only a couple of miles from the Brewery to Nainital climbing almost 3000 feet (915 metres). Everything had to be carried up to Nainital and beyond in this way, on the backs of Indians. Narrelle described their efforts.

> *They look for all the world like gnomes, or, like large beetles on long legs (bare) creeping up the face of the mountain. They carry up everything from a piano to a tin of biscuits, on their backs. They put a rope round the article, & then bring it round their foreheads, & when they want to rest, they back up to the wee stone wall, or the bank, & rest their load on it. Their clothing mostly consists of part of a shirt & a loin cloth.*

At 6500 feet high (1830 metres), Nainital was a pretty hill town in the Kumaon Hills surrounded by miniature lakes, moss-covered boulders, trees and feathery foliage. After six weeks of continuous rain, commonplace in the summer months, the place was completely sodden. Most of the lakes were created over time through landslides, but Narrelle related to her family the Hindu legend pertaining to Nainital which she read about in Jim Corbett's *Naini Tal Guide of 1906*. Her account was taken almost word for word from Corbett's book, a key guide for tourists and travellers at the time.

> *The Hindu legend relating to Naini Tal & the formation of the lake, is that three of the Rishis, or celestial sages (who were created by the great Brahma, & who, later, by reason of their cursing the God Shiva, were by him fixed as the seven stars in the constellation Ursa Major) on their pilgrimage, came by Chitrasila or Ranibagh, to the Gagar range (called after a saint), & ascending the highest peak, China, began a long penance; being in need of water they dug a large hole near the mountain, into which the great god Brahma was pleased to pour waters from lake Mansarowar, the sacred lake in Tibet (we are only about 68 miles* [109 kilometres] *as the crow flies, from Tibet here) & the lake was called Trishisarowar, or the lake of the three Rishis; & ever after anyone who bathed in the lake was purified from sin, even as though he had bathed in Mansarowar itself, oh & then it goes on to tell of the Goddess Narayani Tal, the present name being an abbreviation of this. But it doesn't matter where you go in India, especially in the Himalayas, there is a legend for everything, with their Gods and Goddesses, there is a rock by the edge of the Naini lake, that on festival days is coloured red & around which lights are burnt in honour of the Goddess, even yet, oh they are a wonderful people.*

At Nainital, a reasonably large administrative centre for the British, Narrelle spent a day negotiating with the Indian military and medical authorities, the station staff officer, the medical board, and the *tahsilder*, or 'coolie agent', arranging the next leg of her journey. The quickest and most direct route to Almora and Binsar was over the mountain passes on a pony but Narrelle felt she was not quite well enough to undertake an expedition of that kind. Whilst Narrelle was enjoying this extraordinary journey, it was taxing and demanding on her health, especially as she had not fully recovered. The authorities decided that she had to go back down the mountain to the Brewery by *dandi*, catch a lift in the motorcar carrying the mail to Ranikhet, and then obtain another *dandi* from Ranikhet to Binsar via Almora. So, after three days in rainy Nainital, Narrelle travelled back down to the Brewery by *dandi*. She then caught the car, accompanied by a particularly young junior officer who had just left officer training school at Simla. Off they went

> *… puffing and panting, up, up, up again, great scot how we did go up, looking down thousands of feet over the most wonderful scenery, up into the mts like nothing in Australia, here & there, between gaps catching a glimpse of the hazy plains below, stretching as far as the eye can see, its surface marked here & there by the white lines of one or two quite wide rivers, oh but it was beautiful. Then, rounding one part of a mountain, we came to a road that led down, & away we went, slithering down into the bowels of the earth, so it seemed to Bhowalie. There is a consumptive sanitorium there, also a turpentine distillery. While we were waiting there for the mails to be taken off, we saw a huge motor, gorgeously fitted up, being pushed up the hill by about 40 natives while the driver sat in state, dressed all in white, & I heard some of the natives saying something about 'Maharaja' so came to the conclusion that it was his motor, the Maharaja of Bhowalie. After leaving Bh— we skirted along at the foot of the mountains, along the river bank, for miles. It was intensely hot, & I could feel my cheek on the left side (west) quickly turning a deep brown, & even the colour of my grey frock was gradually changing colour. It was wonderful how the trees and undergrowth changed as we went along, for a time it was absolutely sub-tropical, then after a while the only trees one saw were pine trees, & then the*

mountains seemed to be just bare, with a few small shrubs around ... it was impossible to try & pick out our pathway, either behind or in front, so I gave it up, & gave up trying to think which mountain we would find ourselves on next, phew, looking down over the side of the roads at times, sheer down to the river below, looking like a tiny stream, one came to the conclusion you could have quite a respectable smash up there if anything went wrong with the steering gear, phew — made one quite giddy, to even think of it.

They arrived at Ranikhet around seven o'clock in the evening. Narrelle's accommodation was a 'dak bungalow'.

There are no hotels in most of these little Hill Stations, but there is invariably a dak Bungalow, with a khansamak [a male servant], *who looks after things and either gets meals for you, or cooks your own things, unless you have your own barwarchi (cook), & then he does it, & you simply pay R1 for the use of the room for the night, & of course you have all your own bedding. There is not even a mattress on the bed, but the beds are mostly just wooden frames with wide soft webbing interlaced instead of springs, quite a good idea. The bungalows are generally built on the pick of the town sites, & is of stone, & wide stone verandah & stone posts. I was the only one staying there that night, it was so weird. Ranikhet is a rather pretty place, with a fine view, it's supposed to be one of the healthiest Hill stations in India, and crowds of troops are sent up there during the summer.*

At 8.30 the following morning, Narrelle and her party of nine coolies left Ranikhet. For the next day and a half, they were her only companions. The Indians could speak no English, and Narrelle's Hindustani was very limited, but she had a couple of phrase books with her. Narrelle learnt more Hindustani during that trip than in all her time in Mesopotamia or Bombay. When it was not so steep, Narrelle alighted from her *dandi* and walked using her wooden walking stick purchased in Sicily, always with a coolie trotting behind her carrying her umbrella or Kodak. The weather was incredibly hot, and Narrelle's conscience was pricked by these *poor human horses, it's awful to see the loads they can carry, and for this, they get from annas 4 to 6 a day. A anna is equal to a penny, & there are 16 in a rupee, isn't it awful. I felt an awful pig letting them yank me up some of the mountains, but they go on quite cheerfully.*

They arrived at Almora on dusk, just in time to pay the toll and enter the village. There were tolls on all the small mountain tracks in the Himalayas, and if they had been late, they would have had to camp outside the tollgate. Narrelle was feeling very tired and unwell due to altitude sickness (not surprising as Almora is 5300 feet [1616 metres] above sea level) and her stomach pains had not abated, so they had a late start the following day. Binsar was only 12 miles (19 kilometres) from Almora along a road even more beautiful than the Ranikhet to Almora track. They set off mid-morning, Narrelle walking with her Indian entourage through beautiful scenery. She was mesmerised, transfixed by the mountains towering above, the jungle and large rhododendron trees, begonia and oak trees, the mass of ferns and moss surrounding them, and the valleys way, way, below. Narrelle had read about the leopards and man-eating tigers that terrorised the locals. Her imagination ran wild as she climbed further and further up the mountain path, fuelled by exhilaration and giddiness. The narrow track wound up and around, up and down, all the time climbing higher and higher. Then Narrelle confronted a small herd of water buffalo.

> *On leaving Almora you start & mount up & up. After a bit I got out* [of the dandi] *& walked, on, on we went, ever upwards, till I looked ahead & saw what looked like the top of the mountains, & I heaved a sigh of thankfulness, & said to myself, 'Now we will just have to go down, we can't go up any higher'. But dear me, we simply turned the corner of the jungle, &, lo, another peak to get round. By this time we were so high above the valley below, & the road, not more than 6 feet* [2 metres], *at*

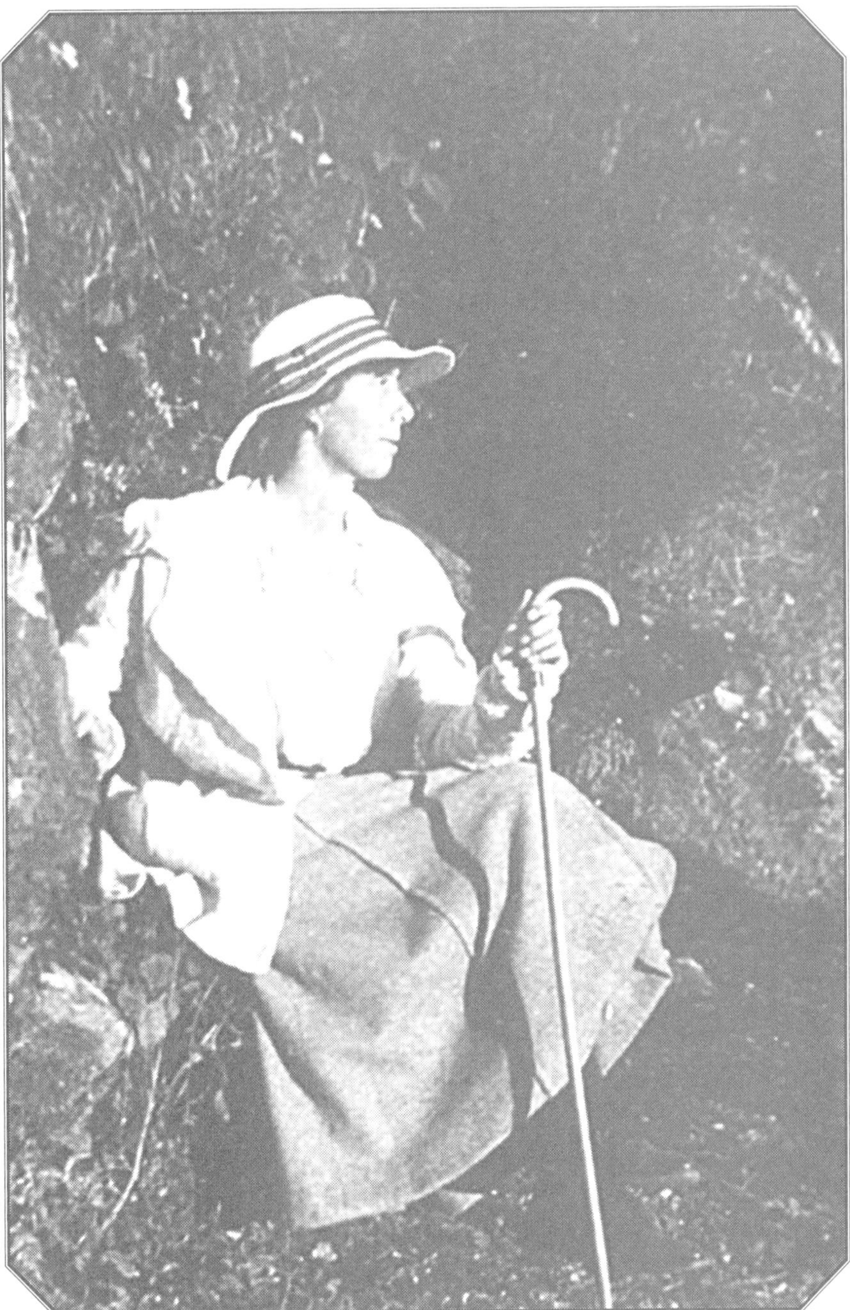

Narrelle with her Sicilian walking stick; Binsar, the Himalayas, 1917. (*Hobbes Collection*)

> *most, wide & no wall, so that as you walked along, the Khud simply slipped away for thousands of feet to the valley below, that after a time I began to get quite giddy as I walked along, & had to get into the dandi. Then at last we got up, & skirted along the top of a mountain, at least I called it a mountain, but I notice they all call them hills, as they are only 8 or 9,000 feet* [2440 or 2745 metres]*!!! Quite molehills, then we began to go down for a few miles, just skirting around, so I started walking once more, & was going serenely on, feeling very proud of myself, having braved the wilds & Himalayas alone with 9 coolies & very little Hindustani, when lo, pride nearly had a real nasty fall. I turned a bend in the road, & there before me I saw a small herd of water buffalo, now if there is one animal in India that I loathe more than another it's a buffalo. I hate their long ugly, evil Hippo looking faces, & their hairless looking black skin like an elephant, & they loathe white people just as much, while a black infant aged 6 can do anything with them.*

Needless to say, Narrelle and her troupe walked safely by past the buffalo, and continued on towards their destination. As they reached Binsar, the clouds and mist rolled in and it began to rain.

NARRELLE'S HOSTS IN BINSAR, THE MARTINS, GREETED THEIR LODGER kindly. An elderly couple who ran a rather ramshackled, run-down farm and orchard estate, they let out rooms for extra income and company. Narrelle described Mr Martin as a *dreamy sort of man* who painted and was *exceedingly nice*, with Mrs Martin as *a most energetic woman* who looked after her in a *most motherly way*. After two years of failed fruit crops due to hailstorms, the Martins relied on providing accommodation to officers and nurses on leave as a main source of income. They had room for six lodgers but Narrelle was their only houseguest. They also rented out bungalows during the summer months. One was occupied by a Mrs Mitchell, whose husband, a major in the Indian army, had recently died in Mesopotamia. The Martins' three sons were also fighting there. One had been killed early in 1917, and another was dangerously ill with enteric fever. Their daughters were married and lived elsewhere. Coincidently, Mrs Martin's siblings lived in Mosman, a suburb close to Cremorne in Sydney where Narrelle's mother and sister lived. Mrs Martin's father had been a judge in India before going to Tasmania. Her sister and nieces were VADs at 'Graythwaite', the grand house donated to the Australian Red Cross by wealthy Sydney businessman Sir Thomas Dibbs as a convalescent hospital, and her brother, Frank Bignold, was a barrister and journalist, who knew Elsie through tennis. It was a small world.

For the first three days it was misty, wet and dull at Binsar. Narrelle stayed indoors, mostly in bed for, not surprisingly, she had found her ten-day journey really exhausting. But early on the fourth morning, the mists disappeared and Narrelle discovered to her amazement that from her private bit of verandah she looked out over the eternal snows, only 30 miles (48 kilometres) away. The sun was shining brightly and she could see straight down into the valley below. She could clearly observe the terraced fields looking like giant steps disappearing down, down, down, all lush and green for as far as the eye could see. And then, all around them were majestic mountains, *purple, blue, green & brown all blending in with the softest haze, & little snowy banks of clouds moving about, now rising, now sinking into the valley with the movement of feathers, wafted about on the highest breeze, there they rose, range upon range till they touched the snow line.*

Narrelle had an unobstructed view.

> *It was the most wonderful & glorious sight I have ever seen. Oh how I wish you could see it all, how you would love it, at times it is almost overpowering in its beauty, there is too much of it, so it seems, but it is a thing to dream of, & I sometimes wonder what I have done ever, to deserve all this pleasure, & I wish I was a better hand at describing things, but somehow it is difficult on paper, but one can never forget it.*

The natives up here have a proverb that runs, somehow like this 'Those who have once lived in Kumaon (this district) & amongst the Himalayas, are never happy elsewhere & must return'.

Narrelle fell ill almost as soon as she arrived. Much to her distress, the stomach pains returned, fast and furious. In such an isolated spot the medical facilities were modest to say the least. The nearest hospital was at Ranikhet, almost 30 miles (48 kilometres) from Almora, but if at all possible, Narrelle did not want to be hospitalised. The medical officer at Binsar was an Indian from one of the regiments, and he, along with two other native Indian doctors' constituted Narrelle's medical board. After examination, they believed Narrelle had a gastric ulcer. They agreed that she could continue to stay on with the Martins, but that she had to go to bed. Mrs Martin agreed to look after her. For the first 36 hours Narrelle was not allowed any food whatsoever, with only sips of hot water when thirsty to prevent dehydration. After that, she was placed on a starvation diet of milk and water, or 'duck's food' as the Martin's son referred to it. This went on for twelve days after which the pain subsided and Narrelle was allowed Horlicks in her milk. The medical board then gave her another six weeks' sick leave up to 25 October when she would again be assessed. There was also the possibility of a further month's leave after that, which Narrelle believed would be *awful* and *disgraceful*. This idea that nurses should not be sick permeated Narrelle's thinking. *That would mean over six months off duty*, she howled to her family. The ignominy of it all did not bear thinking about. Nurses were never meant to get ill. They nursed sick people to health, not the other way round.

So there she was, ensconced at her idyllic hill station, tucked up in bed with blankets and fur rug, a hot water bottle and roaring fire, while observing out of her window the coming signs of winter: the colder, shorter days, the ripening chestnuts, the creepers entwining the deodar and oak trees turning the autumnal colours of yellow, red and brown. By early October, she was still in bed, still on her watered milk diet, largely

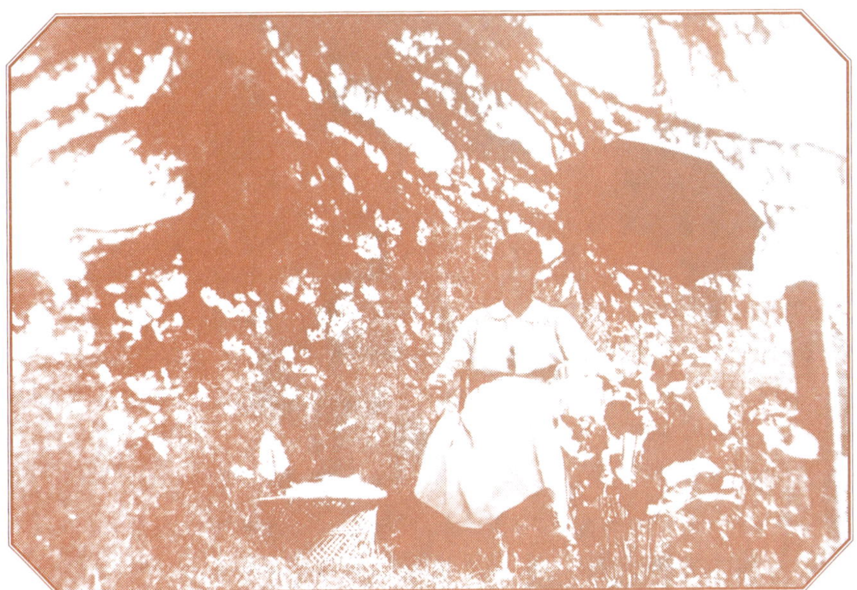

Narrelle under the deodars, Binsar, 1917. This photograph was sent to Frank Webb in France. On the back Narrelle commented, 'Considering I had just had three weeks in bed, on milk only, I guess I don't look too bad…'. (*Webb Collection*)

sleeping. After three weeks, the rain stopped and she sometimes sat outside in her long chair, writing letters and dozing in the sun. Not surprisingly, at Narrelle's next medical board her leave was again extended another month to 6 December.

ONCE SHE WAS SLIGHTLY BETTER, NARRELLE WAS ABLE TO CONTINUE HER beloved activity of writing letters. She moved a little wooden table and chair outside onto the grass, and sat looking towards the magnificent views while she wrote. She used her weekly letters home as a way of overcoming her loneliness. *There is nothing to write about, but it's kind of lonely, so I'll have a chat with the family*, she wrote in a letter addressed to her sister Jean, lovingly referred to as 'old Missus'. Narrelle spilt much ink on the vagaries of the mail system that delivered the precious

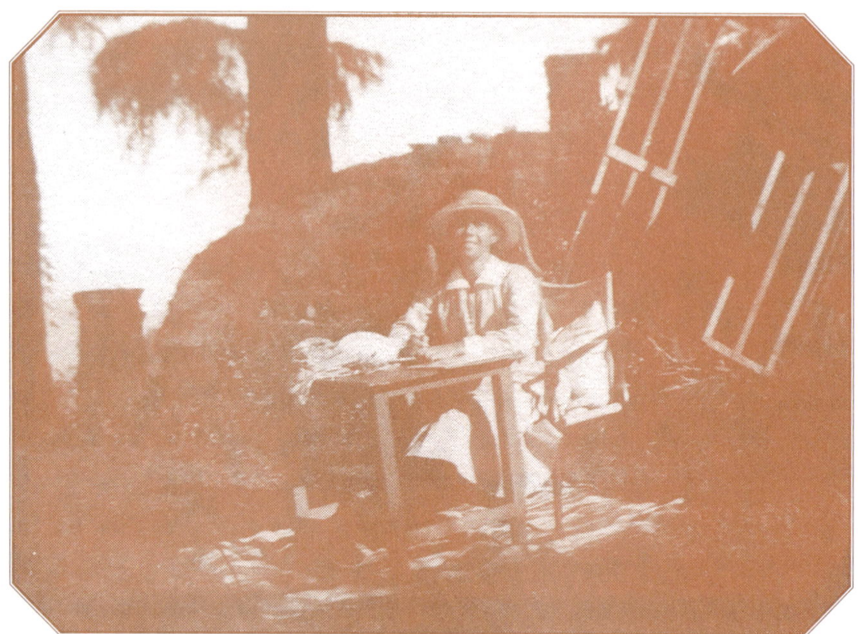

Narrelle writing letters in the sunshine, looking out over the view towards the eternal snows of the Himalayas, Binsar, 1917. (*Hobbes Collection*)

letters, her umbilical cord to the outside world. Her topics of conversation from Binsar generally revolved around her future plans, about getting back on duty, and where she would like to be posted, be it Baghdad, France or Egypt. Much of it was fanciful stuff but Narrelle never gave up the idea of returning to active service. She often mentioned the Martins and asked her mother to write and thank Mrs Martin for all her help. Every night Mrs Martin would come in to Narrelle's bedroom and sit and brush her hair which, with good food and rest, had improved markedly from the Amara days. The women talked quietly about the war, about loss and grief, and the future.

Despite her ill health, or perhaps because of it, Narrelle did not lose her intolerant attitude towards political matters affecting Australia. She continued to comment on the ongoing political turmoil surrounding the second conscription referendum and the Great Strike of 1917. She targeted a family friend for not enlisting.

Those rotters of strikers, I sincerely hope they get conscription, they should have had it long ago, & as for Clem Bate, you can tell him from me, that if his whole body was worth the little finger of one, any one, of the men who are at the front he could be a proud man, as it is I wouldn't give the smallest joint of the smallest finger on any one man of the A.I.F. in Egypt or France, for his whole damned body, or half a dozen of them, the conglomerated rotter, or the pea-eating rotter, I hope I come face to face with him some day, I hope I have a chance to tell him what a skulking coward he is, 'only the rotters are sent to the front' indeed, I boiled so over that bit in your letters my mammy, that I upset my one & only bottle of ink. I would have much pleasure in presenting him with a bouquet of the very, very largest white feathers possible, eugh — but there, he is not worth wasting pencil & paper over.

A main topic of conversation, as always, was the fortunes of her friends, the 'boys' in France, Egypt and Mesopotamia. Narrelle was always thinking of them, wondering what they were doing and how they were coping, if they were safe and well, and not caught up in the fighting. She said that the men in Egypt only received mail every six weeks so she regularly wrote to them with news because she could relate to the longing for news and the counting of the days until the next delivery was due. Holt Hardy was now a lieutenant with the 6th ALH in Palestine, and was a very popular officer with the men. She heard a lovely story from him about Tonie Hordern, also an officer with the Light Horse, who had somehow acquired 42 or so chickens that he had to care for on instructions from the general. Tonie had taken them with him during the Beersheba push, and somehow they survived. Mr Andrews, the Bush Brother from Brewarrina, was wounded in France in late 1917. He was discharged from the AIF field ambulance after the Gallipoli campaign, and became a chaplain with the British army in France. After the war he went to the Sudan to continue his missionary work.

Another young acquaintance, 21-year-old Leslie Dill, a station hand from Brewarrina, was also hurt, again. Like Narrelle's cousin, Gilbert

Anschau, Dill was with the 3rd Battalion, AIF. He was severely wounded for the second time in one year with gunshot wounds to the back, spine and buttocks in April 1917 at Bullecourt in France, and was invalided back to Australia. He was awarded the Military Cross for 'conspicuous gallantry and devotion to duty'. Recovering from his wounds, Leslie Dill returned to the 3rd Battalion as a lieutenant in late 1918. He died during the 1920s.

There was always someone she knew in the wounded and killed-in-action lists. Writing to Kit in late 1917, Narrelle pleaded:

> *Oh Kit if it would only end and let us all go back now, before anyone else is killed. Poor old Ted Nott & Alan & Geoff Yeomans, & crowds of others one knew in those years gone by, there are days when I just get nearly heartbroken at the thought of it all, & the longing to stand on deck & watch Australia come into view. I know I'll yell like a jackal when I do, fancy it will soon be three years since I steamed away, I shall make the Captain tell me what time land should come into sight, & then I'll stay up on deck so as not to miss the first glimpse.*

Much to her distress, Narrelle had not heard from Frank Webb, one of her close friends and regular letter writers, since June. She expected that some of his letters had 'gone down', that is been sunk by submarines or mines. Later in the year she received six letters from him in one week. One had her particularly concerned as Frank mentioned that he was going to try to transfer into the Flying Corps. Narrelle was very perturbed about this because it was so dangerous.

Oh dear I <u>wish</u> he wouldn't, it's a rotten thing, men love it because of the risks they run, because its dangerous, she cried. But then, more philosophically she added, *however, where is it <u>not</u> dangerous these days, even nurses in France are not safe, such a number have been killed lately, working up at the casualty clearing stations, just behind the trenches they can only stand it for about a month at a time.* Frank did not transfer.

When talking about the casualty clearing stations in France, Narrelle was referring to her friends Rose Kirkaldie and Elsie Welman. She kept in touch with the small group of Australian nurses who had sailed together on the *Ballarat* from Australia way back in February 1915. Of the five women, she was the only one still on active service. Rose and Elsie, who served with Narrelle at Malta, were later transferred to France where they worked at a casualty clearing station. Elsie suffered a bad nervous breakdown, or *break up* as Narrelle termed it, and they both returned to Australia. Kath Fitzgerald went home after one year's service, as did Sylvia Bell from Melbourne. Of the men whom Narrelle had met on the *Ballarat*, George Best, was very ill with dysentery in Salonika, and Charlie Cran had been invalided from France, both with Military Crosses; and a couple were still serving in Malta and France.

Narrelle received letters from her colleagues and friends back in Mesopotamia. One of her doctor friends, Maurice Murray, who had been transferred to Baghdad, described the city to her, saying it was much overrated. Quoting from his letters, she related back to her family:

> *'I am afraid I am not much good at descriptions, & I can't explain every thing, bar 2 or 3 mosques & minarets which are really worth seeing, the others are very commonplace all that has been done towards the improvement of the place, was done after we captured it. It is very large, and the type of people here are quite different to those you meet anywhere else in Mesopotamia. Both men & women are most extraordinarily fair, and dress most gorgeously, especially the woman, who are very beautiful in their own way.'*

Narrelle also received letters from Jessie Stow and Thomas Legg, both of whom were transferred to Baghdad in 1917.

One of her special friendships that had developed in Malta was with a patient called George Berrie. He came from Moree and knew Narrelle's brother Charlie, who also lived out there, but Narrelle had never met him in Australia. Narrelle said that he wrote the most interesting letters from the front. She playfully commented that she always enjoyed receiving Holt and Tonie's letters but Berrie's accounts of events such as the evacuation of Gallipoli were really special, beautifully written and so evocative. Berrie recognised his literary potential because after the war he wrote two books about his wartime experiences: *Under Furred Hats*, published in 1919, and later *Morale: A Story of Australian Light Horsemen*. He also wrote a light novella, *Threebrooks*, published in 1934.

George Berrie was closer to Narrelle's age than most of her other friends. He was 33 years old when he enlisted in January 1915 in the second reinforcements of the 6th ALH. A country boy from Forbes in rural New South Wales, he was 6 feet tall with a fair complexion, grey eyes and dark hair. George arrived at Anzac Cove in May 1915, and remained there until admitted to hospital in Malta suffering from debility and colic on 25 August 1915. Narrelle nursed him at St David's Hospital until it was decided to evacuate him to England the following month. He was later reunited with his unit and served in the Middle East, Sinai and Palestine. As with many men, he was promoted up the ranks until becoming a second lieutenant in early 1918.

After three years away, Narrelle missed her family and friends with an aching that simply would not go away. This partly explains why she was so obsessed with nursing and caring for Australian soldiers. They were familiar because they represented home. They spoke the same language. They were, like her, Australian but in a foreign land, working and dealing with foreign people. And the British were the most foreign of all. She tried to explain all this to her sister Kit, tried to explain that that was what motivated her, why she continued to stay on.

> *That's the only reason I would like to be in England for, to see the dear souls when they happen across. It would be such a huge joy, to see a human face I've ever seen before. You simply don't know the feeling, going on for <u>years</u> & never seeing a face you have known before the war. I sometimes wonder if there ever <u>was</u> a time before the war, the only people I've met since leaving Australia, that I'd ever seen before were Tonie*

& Mr Andrews, in Malta two years ago, & then, just before I left Malta for Sicily Geo Berrie turned up, & he knew Charlie, I could have nearly hugged him for having known some of my people, & I'm afraid if any of them turned up now, I should hug them, without the slightest hesitation. However, as they are not at all likely to turn up, there is no fear of my being able to put my threat into practice.

BY NOVEMBER 1917, TWO AND A HALF MONTHS AFTER SHE HAD ARRIVED at Binsar, Narrelle was still having attacks of gastritis. She found sewing a good distraction and was rapidly restocking her supply of undergarments. As she wrote to her mother, *when I have an attack of gastritis, I just lie in a long chair & sew madly all day, it sort of eases the pain*. The medical authorities prescribed a strong bismuth tonic and were cautious in assessing her ability to return to active service. However,

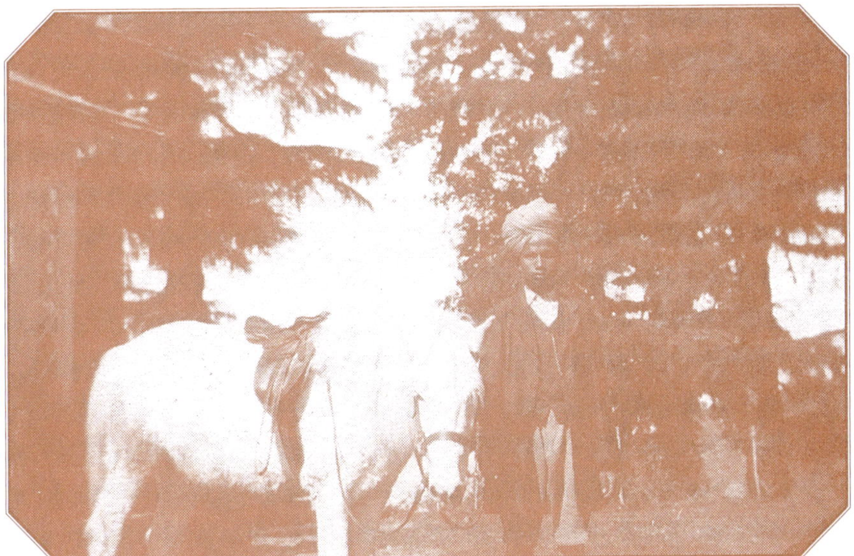

Narrelle's pony, saddled up ready for his charge outside the Martin's house, Binsar, 1917. Being a proficient horse rider, Narrelle occasionally rode when she felt well enough. (*Hobbes Collection*)

despite these spasmodic attacks, Narrelle had put on weight and was happy to stay put in Binsar with the Martins. It was somewhere safe and secure, far away from military life. It was Narrelle's first taste of normality in almost three years.

She fell into the rhythm of life in the hill station. It was very relaxing. The weather was gorgeous with warm and sunny days, and she talked about being as *brown as a berrie*, staying outside all day apart from meal times and bed. The day was structured around meal times and mail deliveries. The maid, or *Chota Hazra* came to Narrelle's room with a cup of tea at 7am, and at eight o'clock brought her bath in. At 10.30, a leisurely breakfast generally continued for about an hour, followed by letter writing as the mail left for Almora at 12.30pm. The incoming mail generally arrived about 2pm, and for the next hour she sat out of the snow wind in the sun, on the lower lawn under the deodar tree reading the mail. At 3pm the tea gong rang. After that a walk was the order of the day either along one of the gentle paths or, if feeling up to it, a climb to the flagstaff on Binsar Hill to watch the sunset.

At over 8000 feet (2440 metres), Binsar Hill was a climb Narrelle tackled only if she was feeling capable, which was not very often. Her walking companion was either Mrs Martin or Mrs Mitchell. These two women, of similar ages, had something in common — Mesopotamia and the war. They chatted quietly about the place as they climbed up to the highest point on Binsar Hill. Narrelle described the scene.

> *From the flagstaff you looked away down the Khud, thousands of feet, to the valley below, and then up, up, over range upon range of the most rugged ranges, bare & golden brown in places, and in others covered with a thick jungle, here & there tucked away on the sunny side, you would see little native villages then up, up, each range getting softer in colour, pale violet & blue, as they neared the snows, then, as you stood facing the snows, as far as the eye could see to the right (east) and the left (north) were these huge, rugged, jagged masses of snows, Nampa in Nepal, & Nanda Kot, Pauch Chule (five fire stalls of the Gods), Nanda Devi,*

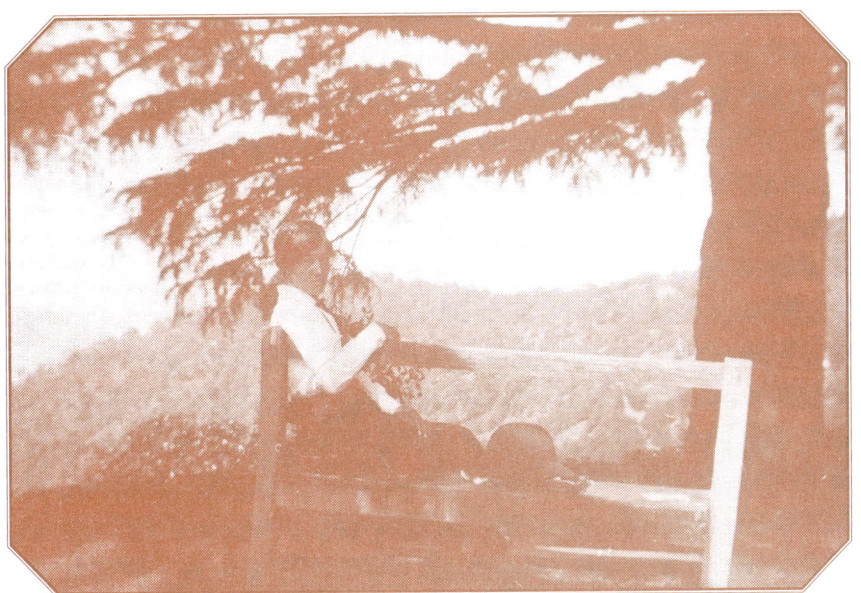

One of Narrelle's walking companions, the recently widowed Mrs Mitchell, Binsar, 1917. (*Hobbes Collection*)

Trisule Dunjairi, Rataban, Mana, Kamat Badrinath, all over 22,000 feet [7826 metres], *& reaching, in the case of Kamet, in Tibet, 29,430* [8976 metres] *& Nanda Devi, 30 miles* [48 kilometres] *away, 25,660* [7826 metres], *& many of them over 23,000 feet* [7015 metres].

At sunset, the sky behind them used to become the most exquisite pink, mauve, shading up into the softest, palest blue, mauve, which again shaded up into the softest, almost duck egg green, then on, getting deeper & deeper, till overhead, it was a deep violet, looking round, into the sunset, the sky was a rich golden pink, while the rays, across the ranges & valleys were like the rays of a rainbow, in purples & red browns, gradually the valley became filled with the most wonderful blue & violet shadows and mists, and a soft purple, almost a pale violet, mist begins to rise up, up, over all the lower ranges, and around the valleys, till they were shaded in the most exquisite, softest violet, through which their darker shades, & massive boulders shone up, and then, above them, & crown of all, turning from the most dazzling white, to the softest shell pink, these towering masses of snow mountains, then, as the sun sinks lower and lower, and the mauve in the sky deepens so also does the colour on the snows deepen and glow, till they seem almost like some living things, perhaps some Goddess of those ancient times, wandering abroad, veiled in the soft mist, as so many of the beautiful Indian women find shelter behind the purdah screen of Indian womanhood — but all too quickly their warm beauty fades, and when at last the sun sinks, a golden ball, behind the ranges of misty purple mountains, in the West, the snow mountains have become white masses, cold, ice blue white against a quickly fading blue mauve sky, and all too soon afterwards, the darkness comes.

Darkness fell about 5pm, and earlier in the winter months of January and February. Due to the prevalence of man-eating tigers and leopards in the forests around Binsar, it was generally considered unsafe to walk around at night unless you had a lantern or were in a group.

IN THE LAST WEEK OF NOVEMBER, DUE TO THE CONTINUOUS ATTACKS OF gastritis, Narrelle was summoned by Major McDonald, the Indian Medical Services' senior medical officer at Almora, for a consultation. He and his wife had only recently transferred from Dehra Dun, a larger town to the north-east that serviced the hill station of Mussorie. On arrival at his new posting, McDonald reviewed his case files, which included Narrelle. He was not happy with what he found, and believed that she may well have to go into hospital for tests and an X-ray to determine the exact cause of her ongoing ill health. He immediately advised her to bring all her kit down from Binsar, and stay with them until her next medical board. Narrelle was unsure of this invitation as she did not know the McDonalds, but the doctor was gently insistent. It was with some reluctance, therefore, that Narrelle packed up her belongings, farewelled the Martins and Binsar, and headed back down the mountain path to Almora.

Chapter 10

'IF ONLY IT WERE TRUE AND THE WAR WAS A THING OF THE PAST'

ON ARRIVAL IN ALMORA, NARRELLE FOUND THE MCDONALDS A *charming* couple in their thirties with no children. He was a rather good-looking man with a cheery disposition, and very interested in his work. He had been serving in Mesopotamia before being invalided to India. Like Mrs Martin before her, Mrs McDonald soon became a firm friend.

After two weeks under Dr McDonald's personal care and medical treatment, Narrelle, again, felt better. He started her on the 'Carlsbad treatment', originally devised by Dr David Becher in the early eighteenth century. This was based on drinking mineral spring water similar to that found in Carlsbad in the Czech Republic. Becher worked out what minerals were in the Carlsbad water, many of which, it was believed, assisted with curing illnesses of the digestive tract, stomach and intestines. People from across Europe trekked to Carlsbad to seek treatment in its spas and waters. In the 1890s, Messrs S. Kutnow and Co from London manufactured Effervescent Carlsbad Powder containing all the ingredients of the famous salts — sodium, calcium, chlorides, sulphates and carbonates — which could be taken by both adults and children. McDonald supervised Narrelle's treatment and combined it with appropriate diet and exercise. As she explained to sister Jean:

I'm doing the 'Carlsbad' treatment, ever since I came in from Binsar, Major McDonald has made me go in for it. Jean my beloved it would do your old liver good too, and is very simple. Get some 'Kutnow' powder and every morning before breakfast — 1 hour — take one teaspoon of Kutnow in a glass of hot water, walking up & down your room all the time you are drinking it, which means that you don't drink it down in one gulp, then stand in the doorway or window, and take deep breathing exercise, for a few minutes, drawing the liver well up & down, it's great, good for the liver. I've done it for a month, solidly, and feel the benefit.

Despite this apparent improvement in Narrelle's as yet undetermined medical condition, her next medical board decided that she should be admitted to hospital for tests and, at McDonald's suggestion, have an X-ray of her stomach and internal organs. McDonald and another doctor stationed at Almora — a woman, Dr Shepard — believed that Narrelle originally had paratyphoid back in June and now had a secondary infection of the gall bladder. *Sounds awful but isn't, quite a usual thing & will be quite all right soon*, Narrelle attempted to reassure her family as cablegrams flew backwards and forwards from Almora to Sydney. McDonald talked of admitting her to hospital at Dehra Dun, where he was previously stationed and where he knew the medical staff well. Dr Shepard's choice of hospital was in the larger city of Lucknow or even Agra, but the military authorities had the final decision. They were to organise Narrelle's papers, including railway pass and road warrants, forthwith.

However, two weeks later, on 17 December, Narrelle wrote to her family in a very angry mood. Nothing had happened. She was very cross with the medical authorities who were incapable, it seemed, of making a very simple decision: *how* was Narrelle to travel from Almora to Kathgodam? The authorities had to sanction the use of a car to transport Narrelle by road, rather than make the three-day journey in a *dandi*. The doctors had firmed up their medical diagnosis; it was one of two things, either gallstones or a paratyphoid infection of the gall bladder. Secondly, they now felt that Lucknow Hospital, despite not being a military hospital, would provide the best treatment. There was also some suggestion of Narrelle being transferred to Nainital, where Major Hunter, a doctor with a great reputation, was based, but that hospital closed in the winter months. Another suggestion was Meerut, the only military hospital in the region. But even though the two doctors had recommended an X-ray, and the medical board had agreed on a hospital stay for Narrelle, little was actually being done to facilitate the suggestion and move forward.

All this delay meant that a return to Mesopotamia and a posting to Baghdad was looking less likely. Narrelle believed the authorities might now send her back to England for military work, an option Narrelle did not like much. Rose Kirkaldie had told her that working in England was awful, 'very stiff' with lots of red tape, something Australians always found hard to take. Narrelle ideally wanted to be posted somewhere where she could nurse Australian soldiers. It is hard to know whether Narrelle was more upset about the apparent indecision of the authorities as regards to her health, or the fact that the delays simply deferred her return to active service. Her isolation, combined with ill health, was making her lose perspective on what was really important: regaining her health as opposed to returning to duty. Her sense of patriotism was becoming misplaced.

There were glimpses of her old self, however, as Narrelle had a well-justified dig at the authorities in charge of her.

> *Well I am still sitting in Almora, and judging from the rapidity!!! with which the Indian Army is moving, I am likely to be sitting here at the end of the war, mis-laid, or still waiting for someone to make a definite statement as to where I am to go, & how. In the meantime I am sitting back enjoying life, at the McDonalds, all the same I could suggest a good big charge of dynamite introduced with some force into the officers of the various doddering A.D.M.S. it's such rot, they seem to think it's some fun letting me dump down on perfect strangers for a month or more.*

Narrelle had been with the McDonalds for over a month and, whilst she enjoyed their company and was feeling better, she could not understand why the authorities were not doing anything. *One of these days I will take things into my own hands, & put my foot down, as much as a mere 'Sister' can in the Army, and tell them they just have to make up their bally vacillating minds, and send me to one place, one time,* she confided irritably to her family.

So it was in Almora, in the depths of the Himalayas, that Narrelle spent her third Christmas on active service. She sent off a small registered parcel with *little tokens of my bestest love to you all, and, just to show you that I haven't quite forgotten you, beloveds.* Despite the high cost of living in India, Narrelle had managed to save up some of her 'field allowance' from working in Mesopotamia so that she could buy a few small presents for her family. Christmas 1917 in Almora was a very quiet affair, apart from officers from the Gurkha regiments singing Christmas carols on Christmas Eve. Narrelle actually wrote letters on Christmas Day and also received a bundle too — the best Christmas present she could have possibly received. As she wrote in a letter:

> *I had a most wonderful & delightful surprise this morning my beloveds. I had just got out of my bath, & doing my hair when, tap, tap, at my door, & a voice in answer to my 'Hah' which means 'Yes' said 'Dak argia (mail is here) Miss Sahib'. I put out my hand, thinking it was probably one letter, from Mrs Martin, as I had got my Australian mail on Saturday, but lo, I had six letters, all from you dear blessed peoples, dated up to 27th Nov — one from Mother, Kit, Josie, Annie & two from Jean, oh it was too delicious.*

If Christmas was quiet, New Year's Eve heralded a dance. Hosted by the officers of a Gurkha regiment in Almora, the whole station attended which meant about twenty women and 30 men. Narrelle did not particularly want to go but the McDonalds persuaded her. At midnight, the bugle called everyone in to the mess room where they had been dancing and the band played 'Auld Lang Syne'.

By New Year, Narrelle was still in Almora with the McDonalds. Judging by the indecision of the army authorities with her case, Narrelle no longer wondered why *they made such an awful mess up of things in Mesopotamia*. The authorities and Major McDonald were busily exchanging letters to each other about Narrelle's condition and what was to happen to her. There was some talk now of sending her straight back to the Colaba Hospital in Bombay. The result of this flurry of correspondence, however, was precisely nothing. *Nothing* was happening. Whilst waiting for the authorities to sanction the use of a car to take Narrelle from Almora to Kathgodam and the train station, McDonald's regime of a diet of fresh eggs, chicken and vegetables, and medicinal treatments appeared to be working. Narrelle said that she was feeling less 'seedy' and much better. Perhaps Major McDonald felt she was responding to his medical care and the urgency of her case had dissipated. Or perhaps the festive season had slowed everything down. Whatever the reasons, it is difficult to understand why there was so little action.

Back in Australia, Narrelle's family was becoming increasingly concerned. Despite her reassurances, they were anxious about her health. Throughout November and December, every time family members met, they could talk of nothing else but what was happening to Narrelle. After much discussion and debate, they decided to act. They had had enough. From such a distance, they could not understand what was going on and why, after six months sick leave, Narrelle was still not well and back on duty. The fact that no proper medical diagnosis had been made also concerned them. What exactly did she have? Why couldn't the doctors work out her illness? Why couldn't she be invalided either to England or preferably back to Australia? Why was she not making more of a fuss? The Narrelle they knew was a feisty, strong-willed woman who would not put up with this treatment. There were just too many questions that letters and the odd cable couldn't answer to their satisfaction from such a distance.

So, over the festive season, they decided on a plan of action. Someone would have to travel to India to ascertain the true extent of her illness. Despite Narrelle's assurances that she was all right, her family, reading between the lines, agreed that affirmative action was overdue. Their mother, at 60 years of age, was too old, and the older sisters had families, children and sick husbands to attend to. So it fell to Elsie, as the youngest sister closest in age to Narrelle, to undertake the trip. Their mother could stay at 'Gunyerwaraldi' or Kit could even come to Sydney with the children if needs be while Elsie was away. The brothers-in-law all put in and paid for her boat passage and agreed on a stipend. Narrelle continually talked about how expensive India was to travel and live in, so Elsie had to have enough money. All they had to do now was get Elsie a passage to Bombay which they quickly achieved. So Elsie Hobbes was despatched to India with a simple mission: to find out exactly what was wrong with Narrelle, and if needs be, bring her back home.

Initially Narrelle was very indignant when she received the cable that Elsie was on her way. She reiterated in a letter dated 14 January that she was recovering and expected to return to duty in February. She argued that there was no great urgency for nurses in Mesopotamia at present and that was partly why the authorities were delaying her return. (This was not true. Nurses were always needed in Mesopotamia but Narrelle was simply not well enough to return to duty).

My dearest peoples,

Darlings, please don't worry about me. I'm quite alright really, and am more fit now than I've ever been for months & months, the absolute rest, & diet & medicine have done wonders and I'm awfully fit, and expect to return to duty about end of February, with luck, I'll be <u>quite</u> fit enough, & if I <u>don't</u> go back then, it will simply be because they are so <u>extra</u> careful, and as Sisters are not so urgently needed up in Mes'pot now, they are in no hurry to send you back, so —

I got a fearful shock when I got your cable on Friday saying that Els was leaving as soon as possible. My dears, she mustn't come, whatever, much as I would love & adore seeing her, but it's much too expensive, and I'm really not ill, and India is a rotten place for a girl to be stranded, unless you've heaps of money. I'm alright, because I've got the Army at my back, & they pay all travelling expenses and messing & everything is so fearfully expensive all the Hotels are £2–10 & £3 a week, alone, it's not like a place where white people predominate, you can't go to a cheap place, because they are only inhabited by natives & Eurasians, and then travelling here is very expensive, unless you are an old hand at the game in India. I find it stiff even tho the Gov pay railway fares & allow you a certain amount for coolies and then it would be very lonely, for if I was in Hospital Els would only be allowed in from 4 to 6, so she must not think of coming. If I was very ill it would be different, but I would probably just be going back to duty, or England, just as she arrived here, which would be too disappointing …

Must stop now darlings. This is only a wee scribble, & I feel it in my bones that it will not go out to you till next English mail comes in, goodness only knows when, unless they have a line just running between India & Aust — anyway I'm chancing it, and please don't worry about me. Oceans of love from Narrie.

As well as despatching Elsie to India, the Hobbes family tried to exert pressure on Australian authorities to negotiate Narrelle's return from India, even if for a short time, to allow her health to fully recover. There was talk of approaching Sir Robert Anderson, Australia's former Department of Defence representative in London who liaised directly with the War Office and General Birdwood on matters of supply, and who had recently returned to Australia. Anderson was a rather controversial figure, whose 'reign at headquarters' according to Charles Bean 'was not altogether a happy one'. Narrelle got wind of her family's idea to pull strings to get her returned to Australia, and responded angrily. She obviously did not think much of the idea or of Anderson.

Josie said something in her last letter about my going back to Australia from here, that they were going to try and fix it up through old Sir Robert Anderson but I've never had any intention of giving up work, as long as I am able to carry on, it's the least one can do for the men who are giving their lives in thousands daily, so long as I am wanted, so long as I am able to carry on. It's my duty to stay where I am, it's no use saying 'but you have done your bit' suppose all the men who have been badly wounded said they didn't see why they should have to go back again, not only once, but again and again, where would the discipline of the army be. Suppose all the sisters who have got ill gave up as soon as they got better, and many of them have been at it since August 1914, who would look after our men, the men who are giving their lives willingly and cheerfully, daily, for us.

If any of you had seen one quarter of the suffering that I've seen during the last three years, or heard the grateful half whispered words of thanks for little things done for them from men, so far spent that they were dependent on you for life itself, and you thought of the wives and mothers of those same men, waiting anxiously at home for news, you wouldn't give them up either. It's the last thing you would think of, dear brave men, they never chose the easiest way. So as soon as I am able, I'm starting right in again, as for that old Anderson man, he may be General Sir Robert but he is nothing but a muddling old fuss box, about as much use to our men over in London as a sick hen and it was a relief to everyone concerned when he went back to Australia, he was a fearful washout could do nothing but think and talk of his own importance as General Sir Robert Anderson, one was always hearing of complaints.

This was more like the Narrelle of old, having a go, opinionated, stubborn, intolerant. And anyway, she argued, the army moves slowly (that was certainly true), and because she was part of the QAIMNS, all her papers and pay had to go through the British War Office in London. It was simply impractical to consider returning to Australia. Furthermore she argued, she had left trunks stored in London and had jewellery and other precious items in safety deposit boxes at the bank in

London, because when they sailed for Malta in April 1915, almost three years ago, all she could take with her was her 'kit'. So, she continued to rationalise to herself and others, she simply could not return to Australia just yet.

ONE CAN CERTAINLY UNDERSTAND NARRELLE'S ATTITUDE TO HER ILLNESS and her increasingly intolerable health situation, and she makes a credible case for carrying on. She is obsessed with war nursing right up until the bitter end. Narrelle identified as one of the boys: she was one of them. *I've been a soldier*, she wrote to her family. Narrelle had developed a peculiar sense of loyalty, a special bond and she would neither betray nor walk away from them. Indeed, she would happily die for them.

> *You know dears, it has never entered my head, or ever will to give up and go back to Australia. I couldn't do it dears, as long as I am wanted by wounded or sick soldiers, and have the health to do it, & I know you would all be the very last ones to want me to, if you had ever seen one quarter of what I have seen our men suffer, or heard the grateful thanks from suffering humanity for the ease & comfort you can give, you perhaps say but there are crowds of women to do it, I say there are not; there are crowds of women eager & willing to don the Kings uniform, & play round, there are more again who have to earn their living & find Army Nursing as good a way as any, & see the world at the expense of the Gov, but alas, there are not very many who have the comfort of their patients at heart, first & last, who are willing to do one extra hour on duty without grumbling.*
>
> *I don't want you to think I am jolly conceited & all that, I'm not, but when, over & over again you hear 'Thank you Sister, it never hurts half as much when you do it', or from some poor half paralyzed soul 'You are good Sister, you always know just how I like my pillows', I ask you, could*

you give them up? Could you slack, & go back to a country that has turned its back on our fighting men, a country that has forgotten — Gallipoli; & the men left there — Never.

I've been a soldier now for nearly three years, & please God I will go right on to the end, as soon as I am fit again, and that won't be very long now, but darlings, as long as I am able to 'carry on' don't, please don't ask me to turn my back on these poor broken bits of humanity, who are dependent upon us, many of them, for life itself, and please remember that, if anything happened, and, I too, passed out, well, there would be no finer way, and no way in which I would be happier, than to lay down one's life for the men who have given everything, and given freely, and suffered as they have, but I guess I'm not doing that for there is much life in this cat yet, so you must not worry about me any, for I am quite all right & happy, & well looked after, and this long rest will just absolutely set me up.

IN THE SECOND WEEK OF JANUARY 1918, NARRELLE WAS STILL AT Almora with the McDonalds. The weather had turned. It was bitterly cold and raining, although Narrelle wished that it would snow. Her temper was finally wearing thin with the Indian medical services and *their vacillating minds, they are too ridiculous*. Narrelle even lost her temper with Major McDonald who, it finally dawned on her, was part of the problem.

I can't say anything about it, for Major McDonald is Indian Army, but he, the old heathen, is as vacillating as any of them, and admits that he hates making up his mind over a thing, they are both most awful dears, but the most thoughtless dear souls possible, perfectly happy just to let things slip along comfortably and not worry about things.

After a couple of gentle reminders, Narrelle finally persuaded the major to send a telegram to Meerut to ascertain her status and their plans for her. She was still upbeat, discussing her future plans, and all the different permutations as to her next appointment, weighing up the pros and cons of serving in Mesopotamia or Bombay. Narrelle even talked about tackling her matron-in-chief, Beatrice Jones, saying that she wanted to be assigned to river transport duty, that she was really due to do that just before she fell ill, that she should have gone to Baghdad instead of India.

Finally, at the end of January 1918, a decision was made. Narrelle was feeling so well — she had gained weight and her colour was good. Major McDonald still wanted her to consult a surgeon to confirm that all was well and that her gallbladder was in good shape, so it was agreed that Narrelle would attend the military hospital at Meerut and then go on to Calcutta, as the hill stations were shutting down because of the winter. The Martins were about to leave Binsar and she could not impose on the McDonalds any longer. Because of her apparent good health, Narrelle was to travel from Almora to Kathgodam by *dandi* rather than car, where she would catch a connecting train to Meerut.

It was with mixed emotions that Narrelle took leave of her mountain retreat, her home for the past three months. On the one hand, she was very sad to leave Binsar and Almora, her refuge, where she had experienced a 'normal' existence, far removed from the exactness and stress of military life. She was also sad to leave her new friends, especially the Martins and McDonalds. But she really wanted to get on with life.

However, the day before she left Almora, she once again felt an *uneasy sort of pain* in her right side. She did not say anything to the McDonalds, who had invited guests over for an evening of dinner and bridge. She somehow excused herself early and went to bed where *the beastly pain came on all over again in fact worse than it had ever been before*. After a sleepless night spent writhing about in pain, she managed to dress and prepare for her journey. The 'acute pain' had worn off but her side was so tender that it was almost unbearable for clothing to touch her stomach. Despite the McDonalds' protestations that she should stay, Narrelle did not want any further delays. She needed to get to a hospital. She had been waiting to leave for weeks. All was in readiness; she must go, sick or not. The coolies were ready and waiting with all her baggage loaded up. Narrelle was loaned a more comfortable *dandi* from one of the local officers' wives with a swing back that allowed her to lie almost flat. Because her military board had decided that Narrelle was well enough to take the *dandi*, not the quicker option of the car, it could not be changed.

Narrelle spent the next two and a half days lying in her *dandi*. Because she was so ill, she did not walk at all, and felt the coolies were rushing her down the mountain path. They had been advised to get her to Kathgodam as quickly as possible, hence their haste. As a result, Narrelle could not take much notice of her surroundings, much to her distress. They went down a different track to the one she was brought up on, to the east of Almora, staying the first night at Peora and the second at Bhimtal, situated around a picturesque lake 5000 feet (1525 metres) up in the mountains. Today Bhimtal, 14 miles (22 kilometres) from Nainital, is a quiet holiday retreat, offering wonderful walks surrounded by terraced citrus farms. On their journey, they passed groups of Tibetans, with flocks of long-haired sheep carrying goods strapped to their back in saddlebags. The Tibetans traded their specialties such as musk pods for rice, dhal and other food. Narrelle's party made it in time to catch the 3pm train from Kathgodam, but she had to change trains three times during the night, which meant little sleep. She arrived exhausted at Meerut the following morning and was immediately admitted to the military hospital. Meerut, only 40 miles (64 kilometres) north-east of Delhi, was a major military centre for the British. It was in stark contrast to the lush, green mountains, and reminded Narrelle of Narrabri or Moree, with its *bare parched plains, wind and dust*.

Narrelle was immediately examined by a surgeon. He decided to send her directly on to Bombay for specialist treatment and advised Narrelle that she would probably have to have an operation to remove a gallstone and drain the gallbladder. But still no diagnoses. Despite the urgency of Narrelle's case, it took a couple of weeks for the travel plans to be made. In the meantime, Narrelle lay in her hospital bed writing letters home — *I seem to have spilt a lot of pencil over these sheets and all about nothing* — with occasional visits by nursing staff when off duty and the chaplain who sent her a bunch of roses every day. They reminded her

> *... of my dear Australian man in Malta. I had an awfully bad cold and Matron made me stay in bed and this man got out of Hospital and walked all the way in to Valletta and out again because he had spent his remaining money on a huge bunch of roses for me. A sister brought them up to me and said 'Sister I just met an Australian soldier who gave me these and asked me to give them to you' and tied on the end was a tiny slip of paper with 'From Peter' on it. He was invalided back to Australia, and has I think died, since, poor boy, do you wonder that I want to start right in again as soon as ever I can get going.*

Narrelle finally travelled to Bombay with another sister, Miss Montgomery, or Montie as Narrelle called her, an Indian Service Sister who had contracted meningitis and was very sick. She was being invalided back to England. Montie could hardly walk, so needed assistance the whole way. The two sick sisters were accompanied by a 'Terrier', or Territorial Sister, who looked after them. The matron organised a whole carriage for the three women, so they *travelled in the lap of luxury*, complete with their own bathroom and large white bath. Farewelled by the staff, the train left Meerut at six o'clock in the morning, bound for Delhi. After only a three-quarter hour stop in the capital, they continued on towards Bombay.

Again Narrelle travelled across the plains of Rajasthan. Once again they reminded her of Australia, only this time the plains were parched, dry, brown and bare, with wind and dust storms and a smoky heat haze, just like the plains of western New South Wales in a drought or dry spell. Wrapped in warm coats and hugging hot water bottles at Meerut, they gradually discarded the warm clothing, so by the time they reached Bombay at 1pm the following day, they were once more feeling the effects of the warm Indian climate.

By 19 February 1918, Narrelle was again ensconced at the Colaba War Hospital being looked after by five *cheery Australian Sisters* all from Tasmania and Victoria. She was so excited to think that Elsie was on her way. To see her after all this time was almost too much to bear. She ticked off the days like a child waiting for Christmas and Santa Claus. She had put all her earlier concerns about money and cost to one side. It would be so good to see Elsie, to see her beloved sister, someone from home.

On her arrival at the hospital, Narrelle underwent a series of tests and X-rays. She was finally having the X-rays that Major McDonald had suggested three months earlier. Over three days, Narrelle's stomach was filled with bismuth, bread and milk for the tests. The doctors were looking for ulcers, gallstones, indeed any abnormal growths or tumours to ascertain the cause of her ongoing illness. On 24 February, Narrelle was wheeled into theatre for an operation.

Going Home

Chapter 11

'THE LONGING TO STAND ON DECK & WATCH AUSTRALIA COME INTO VIEW'

ELSIE SAILED FROM SYDNEY TO SINGAPORE ON THE *MATARAM*, WHERE she was held up by a cyclone. Frustratingly she had to cool her heels in Singapore to wait out the storm. There Elsie received a cable from the hospital asking her arrival date and urging her to get to Bombay as soon as possible. The news was not good and she feared the worst. Finally the cyclone abated and the second leg of Elsie's journey began. She sailed up the Straits of Malacca, dog-legged around the Nicobar Islands, and set course directly across the Indian Ocean to Madras on the east coast of southern India. She arrived at the bustling Indian port around 2 March, two weeks after Narrelle's operation. From there, it was a long train journey northwards across the subcontinent to Bombay. Met at the train station by a nurse from the Colaba War Hospital, Elsie did not have to negotiate the frantic transport options in the foreign city and, after collecting her belongings, together they hurried out to the hospital on the outskirts of Bombay.

Elsie was taken to the matron and quietly told of her sister's condition. It was important to prepare her before she saw Narrelle. The operation had not been a success. Narrelle had advanced liver cancer. She was dying.

Elsie was warned that Narrelle was extremely weak, could barely sit up, and spent much of her day sleeping. She was on morphine to ease the pain. Elsie was also informed that preparations were being made to send Narrelle immediately back to Australia. The quickest way was to transport her to Colombo by train and then take a hospital ship home. But the train journey took five days and four nights, and the doctors did not think Narrelle was capable of enduring such a lengthy train trip as she was so desperately ill. The alternative was to wait for the Australian hospital ship *Kanowna*, due to arrive in Bombay in a few days' time. The ship was on her way to Egypt via Aden and Suez to pick up patients in Alexandria, and then would return to Australia.

Elsie tried to absorb all this information as she was escorted through the hospital complex to the Nurses' Hospital. Narrelle was in a room of her own. It was fairly nondescript, not large, painted white, with a bed, locker, two visitors' chairs, and a bedside table covered in flowers. What it did have was a small balcony which looked out over the rose garden, with doors open to catch the breeze. Narrelle was asleep, breathing lightly. She looked peaceful, pale and gaunt. Elsie caught her breath and hesitated before tiptoeing into the room and taking one of the chairs. Placing her handbag carefully on the floor beside her, not wishing to wake Narrelle, she perched on the edge of the chair, crossing her ankles underneath for support. She sat, absolutely still, for perhaps ten minutes, just looking at her sister. A bunch of bedraggled wattle so carefully wrapped up in brown paper, and brought to remind Narrelle of home, remained in her lap. Elsie then slowly placed her hand in Narrelle's, and leant over her and kissed her on the cheek. Narrelle's eyes flickered open and she smiled. 'I've been waiting and waiting for you, Els. At last.'

'I'm here to take you home,' said Elsie softly. 'I'm here to take you home.'

Matron organised for Elsie to stay in the nurses' quarters at the Colaba to be closer to her sister, rather than hiking back into town and staying in a hotel. Everyone was very kind and helpful. Elsie's arrival perked Narrelle up and she even managed to write a short letter home to her mother on 20 March where she warned that, *I will have to go straight into Hospital on arrival in Sydney dears, so don't expect me to look awfully well, as the trip will probably upset me a bit, but I'll have Els with me, such a joy.*

Narrelle's last letter was written from Suez on 11 April 1918.

My darlings,

Just a wee note today as they have just told me a ship is going out, & I made Els go up to Cairo with some of the girls, I know she will love it, & it would have been too bad to come to Suez & not go on & see Cairo. She didn't want to go at first, she didn't want to leave me, but I told her I wanted her to go, it's the chance of a lifetime.

We had a fairly good trip over, I had two or three rather bad days, but that was only to be expected. The weather is wonderful, beautifully cool, & at nights we have to use blankets, even here at Suez, such a treat.

We've some awful dears of Sisters on ship, especially the one looking after us.

Oh, the stinks of Suez really they are dreadful. Thank goodness when we at last turn Southwards, the days will all be too long. You know dears I'm horridly ill yet, can't improve at all, it's so beastly, & I really have a beastly lot of pain, & get so tired of it at times, & feel I can't battle against it for an awfully long time, it may improve as we get into the cooler climate, I hope so.

I'm so glad Els has had this chance of seeing Cairo.

Then we call in at Colombo on our way back, 12 days to Colombo, 12 to Perth, then on, cheers — Must stop now dears I can't write much at a time & Matron is going ashore.

Oceans & tons of love to you all from

Narrie.

This was the eighth voyage of the SS *Kanowna*. She had left Sydney on 27 February 1918 under the stewardship of Captain Gilling after a short dispute with the crew over union labour, which delayed departure by a day. The unionist firemen refused to sail until ten other non-unionist crew were replaced. Not to encourage any undue delays, the captain acquiesced to the demand and new unionised crew were sought. The medical staff included AANS nurses and orderlies under the charge of Matron Ethel Strickland and AAMC doctor Lieutenant Colonel Archibald Brockway.

Not surprisingly, there was always a full compliment on these return journeys from Alexandria, and this voyage was no different. The patients were AIF men invalided home for a variety of medical reasons, with some in better health than others. Sometimes the patients did not make it home and were buried at sea. Four AIF men died on this trip. After leaving Egypt on 15 April 1918, there were two funerals as the *Kanowna* sailed down the Red Sea, through the Gulf of Aden, and out into the Indian Ocean. Private Alfred George Chapman, aged twenty, died on 18 April, followed by 31-year-old Second Corporal C.J. Hoyes, 6th Battalion AIF on 21 April. After stopping at Colombo, the *Kanowna* crossed the equator on 3 May but there was little to celebrate. Sister N. Hobbes and a couple of other patients were seriously ill.

On the evening of 9 May, at 6pm, Private Harry Reid died. The 31-year-old rabbit trapper from Bendigo in Victoria had enlisted in June 1916 in the 38th Battalion. From June to October 1917, he was wounded three times. First he suffered shrapnel wounds at the Battle of Messines, then a gunshot wound to the back in July, and at Ypres, on the 12 October, he received a gunshot wound to the chest which shattered his ribs and lungs. An unmarried man, he left his worldly possessions, which were not much, to his friends Levi and Martha Bennett, farmers from Knowsley, near Bendigo.

Narrelle Hobbes died the following day, at ten o'clock in the morning, on 10 May 1918. She was 39 years old. The engines were slowed, and after a simple funeral service led by the Church of England chaplain, she was buried at sea, four days out from Fremantle and Australian soil. Jessie Stow's premonition two years earlier that Narrelle had died and was buried at sea had come true.

The grief experienced by Elsie Hobbes at that lonely funeral and during the final weeks on board ship was so profound that she never spoke of Narrelle's last days, and never spoke of her death or referred to it in any way afterwards. She sent a simple cable to her family announcing the passing of their beloved sister, and nothing more. She knew the military would do the same. Elsie felt responsible for Narrelle's death; she felt that she had failed her family and her dying sister. Narrelle's death cast a long shadow over the Hobbes family for many years. Like so many other Australian families during World War I, they had to deal with the death of a loved one on the other side of the world, many, many miles from home — although in Narrelle's case, she nearly made it home.

Although a condolence letter was sent to Mrs Hobbes on behalf of the king and queen in November 1918 after the armistice, it took time for the relevant authorities to settle the paperwork. Because Narrelle had enlisted with the QAIMNS, yet was an Australian and died on an Australian hospital ship, it took months to finalise details of her pay and war gratuity that Narrelle had willed to Elsie, as the last unmarried sister. Elsie spent years tying up the loose ends of Narrelle's war service. She had possessions scattered all over the place, with trunks and valuables stored in London as well as her kit from India. Because Elsie was so distraught on the *Kanowna* after Narrelle's death, it took her some time to track down her trunks containing precious papers and other personal effects.

It took the War Office almost a year to issue a death certificate, required for probate and other legal reasons. The Hobbes family's solicitors finally received official notification from the British in February 1919.

Narrelle's death made Elsie restless. In 1921 she married an Englishman, John Thorburn, and went to live in Burma and later England. She rarely returned to Australia and died in England in July 1947.

In June 1918, a huge memorial service was held at St Paul's Cathedral in London for nurses who had fallen during the war. The service, led by Queen Alexandra and her daughters, was attended by upwards of 5000 nurses from the QAIMNS; the VADs; and the American, Australian, South African, New Zealand and Canadian services. The service consisted of hymns, the dead march played by the Coldstream Guards, and the last post. Three hundred and fifty names were listed on a Roll of Honour at the service. This included nurses who had died of wounds — the result of bombings of hospitals and casualty clearing stations — from diseases contracted from patients, and the many who had drowned after ships were torpedoed. Others died from being physically and mentally overcome by their wartime nursing experiences.

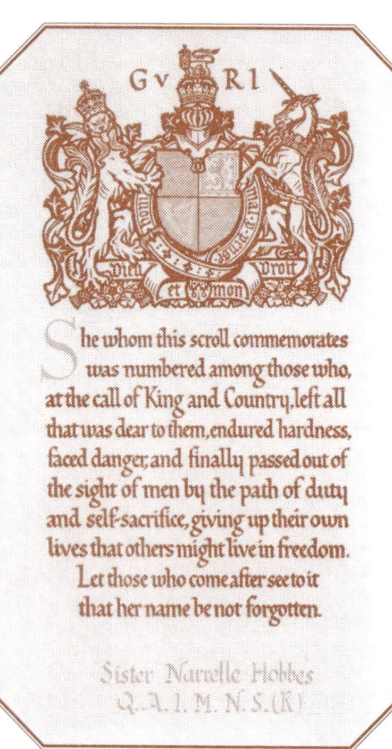

G v R I

Dieu et mon Droit

She whom this scroll commemorates was numbered among those who, at the call of King and Country, left all that was dear to them, endured hardness, faced danger, and finally passed out of the sight of men by the path of duty and self-sacrifice, giving up their own lives that others might live in freedom.
Let those who come after see to it that her name be not forgotten.

Sister Narrelle Hobbes
Q.A.I.M.N.S.(R)

This memorial scroll, which includes the emblem of George V, was given to the next-of-kin of British soldiers and nurses who died on active service during World War I. (*Hobbes Collection*)

Narrelle's name is not listed at the Australian War Memorial because she did not enlist with the Australian nursing service. But her name can be found near the beautiful stained-glass window in York Minster, England, dedicated in the 1920s, which commemorates all British and Commonwealth nurses who died in World War I. And her name was also etched into panel 43 of the Basra War Memorial, her last official posting and from where she was invalided in June 1917. This memorial was relocated by Saddam Hussein in the 1990s and, according to the Commonwealth War Graves Commission, its current state is uncertain. Narrelle was also mentioned on the 'Weilmoringle' Honour Roll, now held by the Brewarrina Historical Society. Of the fifteen names listed on the roll, five have crosses against them, one of them Narrelle's.

The Hobbes family also memorialised their sister. Isabel, the eldest sister who lived in Pymble, renamed her weatherboard cottage 'Narrelle'. On the stone gates she placed a bronze plaque with her name etched into it, as a constant reminder for them all. Her husband, Donald Commons, was later asked by Ku-ring-gai Council if their street could be named after a fallen soldier, a common practice in the aftermath of the war. Despite the misspelling, it was renamed 'Narelle Avenue', in honour of Narrelle Hobbes, and continues to be called that today.

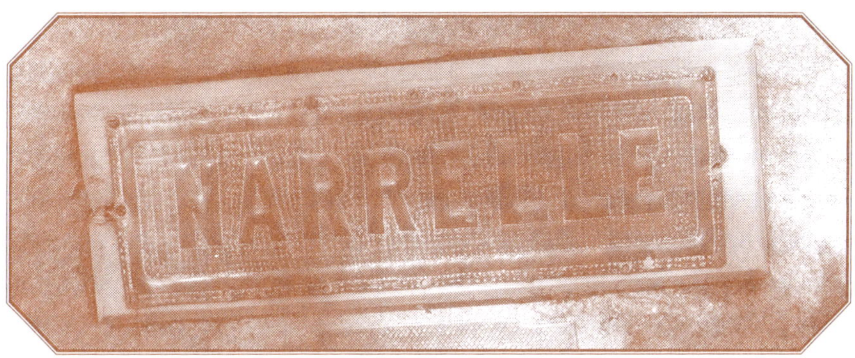

IN CONCLUSION LET US RETURN TO THAT INFORMAL TENNIS GAME AT 'Weilmoringle' in 1914. All of the young men pictured in the photograph enlisted in the war, including Narrelle, the probable photographer. They all returned home safely, with the exception of Narrelle. Holt Hardy, one of Narrelle's special friends, was the first to enlist on 11 September 1914 in the 6th ALH. He landed on Gallipoli on 20 May and managed to stay there without getting wounded or sick — a remarkable feat — and was evacuated at 10pm on 19 December. He was promoted from trooper to captain during the war, was awarded the Military Cross in 1918, and returned home in 1919. Holt remained a bachelor for years afterwards, marrying in his forties. He died on 3 July 1975.

Next to enlist was Roland Bret Allport, known as Bret. He enlisted in the 3rd Battalion, 6th Reinforcements on 11 May 1915. Less than three months later he was on Gallipoli. Bret had a horrendous war. He was wounded at Gallipoli (shrapnel wounds to the head) during the Battle for Lone Pine but survived after months in 1st AGH at Heliopolis. After returning to duty, he was transferred to France, where he was promoted to second lieutenant in August 1916. A week later at Pozières, he was severely wounded, receiving shrapnel wounds to his chest and right leg below the knee, as well as a gunshot wound to the cheek. After extensive medical treatment in England, in which shrapnel was left embedded in his leg, he returned, again, to France, and was wounded again, at Passchendaele in October 1917. This time he received gunshot wounds to his right eye and jaw, left leg, right shoulder and chest. Not surprisingly, having survived three of the worst battles in Australian military history, Bret was invalided back to Australia in November 1917, and was discharged from the army six months later. He never really recovered from his wounds and died eighteen years later, on 13 March 1936. He was 42 years old.

The last two men in the photograph sitting on the right were friends Frank Webb and James Langwell. They were the last of the group to enlist, joining up together in September 1915. From his service record, Langwell was promoted to sergeant, and had a fairly uneventful and safe war. Frank was wounded once in 1917 but, like James, was promoted and returned safely to Australia in June 1919 on the *Runic*. Frank Webb returned to 'Weilmoringle' and became the manager. He married Airini Thompson, a friend of the Hobbes family, in 1923. Frank, Holt and

Tonie Hordern all remained friends after the war, going into partnership with each other and purchasing properties in the Brewarrina area.

As Erich Maria Remarque wrote in his classic *All Quiet on the Western Front*, 'they were part of a generation that was destroyed by the war even those who survived the shelling'. Each of these young people had a story to tell. Each story was different. They belonged to an Australia that we no longer recognise, a time that has well and truly passed. Yet, 90 years on, their war legacy is as important to Australians as ever. We owe it to the men and their memory, but we also owe it to the women — the nurses, including those like Narrelle Hobbes, who served, and paid the ultimate price — to remember their war service alongside that of the boys, for their stories are just as interesting, just as moving, and just as important.

Narrelle Hobbes' war provides us with another lens through which to view Australia's involvement in World War I. Her story further enriches our understanding of that global conflict, and reinforces the fact that Australian women actively participated, nursed, travelled, and sometimes sacrificed their lives for their country.

Let those who come after see to it
That her name be not forgotten.

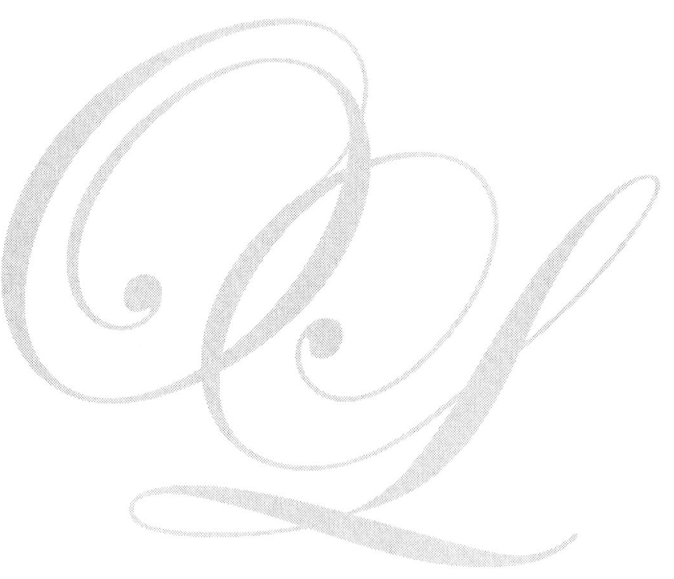

Notes on Sources

The main collection of letters of Narrelle Hobbes is held at the Australian War Memorial, 2DRL/0162. These letters were deposited by Narrelle's mother, Margaret Hobbes, in the early 1930s, with assistance from Eleanor MacKinnon. The collection includes two 'books' of letters from London and Malta, 1915–1916, and Mesopotamia, 1916–1917. It also includes some official correspondence such as the War Office telegrams and commemorative scroll.

The other main collection is held by Rona MacKay and includes two 'books' of letters from Sicily and Bombay, 1915–1916, and the Himalayas up until Narrelle's death, 1917–1918. There are also additional letters from Betty Hall and Tina Withers-Payne, and a small black notebook and photograph album from which many of the illustrations come. On completion of the book, all these papers will be donated to the AWM to supplement their existing lengthy collection.

There are also photocopies of about twenty letters of Narrelle's in the Joan Kingsley-Strack Papers, MS 9551, National Library of Australia, Canberra. These are mainly, but not all, typed copies of letters already held in the AWM.

Other archival sources for Narrelle Hobbes are:

- 'Hobbes N (Sister) — Queen Alexandra's Imperial Nursing Service Reserve — died at sea 10 May 1918', MT1487/1 2001/00494397, National Archives of Australia, Canberra.

- 'Narrelle Hobbes', AWM93 12/1 1/3089.

- War Office: Directorate of Army Medical Services & Territorial Force. Nursing Service Records, First World War, Narrelle Hobbes WO399/3867, National Archives, Kew, UK.

For information about the Hobbs/Hobbes family, see personal communication with Dr Victoria Haskins about aspects of her family history, held by author; additional information supplied by Rona MacKay and Mary Hazelton, held by author; JT Hobbs' diary deposited in Morgan Library, New York; Les G. Thorne, *A History of North Shore Sydney. From 1788 to Today* (Sydney, 1970); Merri Gill, *Weilmoringle* (Dubbo, c. 1996).

For a detailed history of Joan Kingsley-Strack (née Commons) and her work, see the book *One Bright Spot* (Basingstoke, 2005) beautifully written by her great-granddaughter and historian, Dr Victoria Haskins.

For a history of nursing, the AANS and QAIMNS, see Anne Summers, *Angels and Citizens: British Women as Military Nurses* (London, 1988); Elizabeth Haldane, *The British Nurse in Peace and War* (London, 1923); May Tilton, *Grey Battalion* (Sydney, 1933); Lyn Macdonald, *The Roses of No Man's Land* (Ringwood, 1980); Marianne Barker, *Nightingales in the Mud* (Sydney, 1989); Jan Bassett, *Guns and Brooches. Australian Army Nursing from the Boer War to the Gulf War* (Melbourne, 1992); Margaret R. Higonnet (ed.), *Nurses at the Front. Writing the Wounds of the Great War* (Boston, 2001); Juliet Piggott, *Queen Alexandra's Royal Army Nursing Corps* (London, 1990); Ian Hay, *One Hundred Years of Army Nursing* (London, 1953).

See also the *Australasian Nurses' Journal*, various issues from 1914–1920 and Australasian Trained Nurses' Association, Records, 1899–1976, MLMSS4144, Mitchell Library, Sydney.

For Malta during World War I see R.A. Kirkcaldie, *In Grey and Scarlet* (Melbourne, 1922); Rev. A. Mackinnon, *Malta: The Nurse of the Mediterranean* (1916); British Red Cross Society, *Reports by Joint War Committee* (1921); W.G. Macpherson, *Medical Services General History, Vol. 1* (London, 1921); 'Hospitals of Malta', *The Australasian Nurses' Journal*, vol. XIII, No. 12, 15 December 1915, pp. 436–437.

For general descriptions of the AIF see Michael Tyquin, *Gallipoli. The Medical War* (Sydney, 1993); Peter Cochrane, *Australians at War* (Sydney, 2001); C.E.W. Bean, *The Official History of Australia in the War of 1914–1918, volume II, The Story of ANZAC* (St Lucia, 1981 [1924]);

Melanie Oppenheimer, *All Work No Pay* (Walcha, 2002); Bill Gammage, *The Broken Years* (Canberra, 1974).

World War I soldiers' service records are held in the National Archives of Australia, Canberra in series number B2455. The following soldiers records were accessed: Allport, Roland Bret; Anschau, Gilbert Goldie; Andrews, Leonard; Barton, Maurice Darvall Edward; Berrie, George Lachlan; Chateau, Rex Muller; Chapman, Alfred George; Cooper, Gordon Colin; Cutts, Robert Charles; De Garis, Ralph Edwin; Glennie, Charles Oswald Stuart; Dill, Herbert Leslie; Hamilton, John Helenus Scott; Hardy, Holt; Hartridge, Wilfrid; Hobbs, Kenneth Charles Stuart; Hobbs, Reginald Thomas; Hordern, Cecil Anthony; Hoyes, Ormond James; Langwell, James; MacKinnon, Roger Robert Addison; Reid, Harry; Smith, Colin; Solling, Rex Aubrey Fritz; Waugh, Keith Cameron; Yeomans, Geoffrey Heron; Yeomans, Sydney Ernest; Webb, Frank; Worth, William.

Commonwealth War Graves Commission, www.cwgc.org lists casualty details. The following records were accessed: Nott, E.R.; Hartridge, Herbert Wilfrid; Yeomans, Geoffrey; Glennie, Charles Oswald Stuart; Anschau, Gilbert Goldie.

Australian Red Cross Wounded and Missing Enquiry Bureau files, I DRL/0428, AWM, Canberra. File of Gilbert Goldie Anscheu, 0110702.

Worth Family Papers, MS 6980, are held in the Mitchell Library, Sydney. William's wife, Joan Butler, was a cousin of Charles Bean, the Australian journalist, historian and founder of the AWM.

For Tonie Hordern, see Lesley Hordern, *Children of One Family: the Story of Anthony and Ann Hordern and their descendants in Australia* (Sydney, 1985); see also George Berrie, *Morale: A Story of Australian Light Horsemen* (Sydney, 1949).

For Sicily in World War I, see Norma Lorimer, *By the Waters of Sicily* (London, 1901); Norma Lorimer, *On Etna* (London, 1918); Douglas Sladen and Norma Lorimer, *Queer Things about Sicily* (London, 1905).

For a history of the Mesopotamian campaign, see F.J. Moberley, *Official History of the War. Mesopotamia Campaign, 1914–1918, volume 1*

(London, 1923); W.G. Macpherson, *Official History of the War. Medical Services, Diseases of the War, 2 volumes* (London, 1922–23); W.G. Macpherson, *Medical Services. General History, volume IV*, (London, 1924); 'Hospitals in Mesopotamia', *The Australasian Nurses' Journal*, vol. XV, no. 4, 16 April 1917, pp. 133–135; 'Hospital Ship Work in Mesopotamia', *The Australasian Nurses' Journal*, vol. XV, no. 7, 16 July, 1917, pp. 234–236; K. Burke (ed), *With Horse and Morse in Mesopotamia* (Sydney, 1927); A.J. Barker, *Neglected War: Mesopotamia*, 1914-1918 (London, 1967).

See also 'The Last Post. 5,000 Nurses in St. Paul's. Women's Memorial Service', *Australasian Nurses' Journal*, vol. XVI, no. 7, 15 July 1918, pp. 219–220; *The Nursing Record*, various issues.

INDEX